AN INVESTIGATION INTO THE
PRINCIPLES OF HEALTH VISITING

COUNCIL FOR THE EDUCATION
AND TRAINING OF HEALTH VISITORS

First published in 1977

ISBN 0 906144 00 0

Published by The Council for the Education and Training of Health Visitors,
Clifton House,
Euston Road,
London,
NW1 2RS

Printed in Great Britain in Photon Times New Roman
by The Whitefriars Press Limited,
London and Tonbridge.

Foreword

This Report is the result of studies which were stimulated by the annual conference of Health Visitor Tutors held at Wansfell in 1974 and it was drawn up by a Working Group which reported to the Education Committee of the Council in the summer of 1977. Although it was initiated by those engaged in teaching Health Visitors and was presented to the Statutory Body responsible for the education and training of Health Visitors, contributions to the study were made by many Health Visitors and Nursing Officers actively engaged in the Health Visiting Service.

Even though the Report is the result of the deliberations of a Working Group and is not therefore in any way a policy statement, nevertheless the Council is of the unanimous opinion that the material it contains is of such value that it should be published in its entirety to provide information and the opportunity for discussion and debate in the belief that the thinking it embodies can form the basis for new initiatives in the future.

The Council, therefore, would very much welcome comments and observations on this document.

Chairman,
Council for the Education and
Training of Health Visitors.

The Council wishes to record its appreciation of the contributions made by all those who were involved in the discussions and in the compilation of the Report, and especially to the following members of the Working Group:

Miss S. A. Jack (Chairman)
Principal Lecturer in Community Health Studies, Polytechnic of the South Bank.

Miss H. J. Ash
Senior Lecturer in Health Visiting, North Gloucestershire College of Technology.

Miss R. A. Burton
Senior Lecturer in Health Visiting, Huddersfield Polytechnic.

Miss S. G. Campbell
Senior Lecturer in Health Visiting, Ulster College, The Northern Ireland Polytechnic.

Miss L. M. Capel
Senior Lecturer in Health Visiting, Leicester Polytechnic.

Miss P. R. Hay
Professional Adviser, Council for the Education and Training of Health Visitors.

Miss A. Jameson
Professional Adviser, Council for the Education and Training of Health Visitors.

Miss M. McClymont
Principal Lecturer in Health Visiting, Stevenage College of Further Education.

Miss F. Welch
Senior Lecturer in Health Visiting, The Welsh National School of Medicine, Cardiff.

Mrs. M. White
Senior Nursing Officer (Community), Merton, Sutton & Wandsworth Area Health Authority.

Miss H. M. Williams
Principal Lecturer in Health Visiting, Trent Polytechnic, Nottingham.

Mrs. C. T. Wilson
Principal Lecturer in Social Policy and Social Administration, North East London Polytechnic.

The Council would also like to express its thanks to Miss Ruth Schröck whose help in providing philosophical guidance was invaluable.

Contents

		Page
FOREWORD		3
CHAPTER 1	INTRODUCTION	7
CHAPTER 2	THE DEVELOPMENT OF A PROFESSION	11
CHAPTER 3	HEALTH AS A VALUE	20
CHAPTER 4	THE SEARCH FOR HEALTH NEEDS	26
CHAPTER 5	STIMULATION OF THE AWARENESS OF HEALTH NEEDS	34
CHAPTER 6	THE INFLUENCE ON POLICIES AFFECTING HEALTH	44
CHAPTER 7	THE FACILITATION OF HEALTH-ENHANCING ACTIVITIES	53
CHAPTER 8	FURTHER ISSUES	59
APPENDIX I	THE PARTICIPATIVE PROCESS	64
APPENDIX II	THE PROCESS OF RE-APPRAISAL	67

Chapter 1

Introduction

The profession has reached a stage where in order to develop further it must spell out its implicit principles which ultimately predict and guide its practice.

1.1 The Council for the Education and Training of Health Visitors (C.E.T.H.V.) became aware of the need to revise the syllabus following one of its annual conferences for tutors, held at Wansfell in 1974, at which the subject discussed was Section Five of the Syllabus 'The Principles and Practice of Health Visiting'. The main concern was that the principles, which were defined in ethical terms, no longer appeared adequate to describe the process of health visiting. Over the last decade rapidly changing health and social conditions had led to the introduction of new legislation and new patterns of working and to changing consumer expectations. These changes had affected the functions of the health visitor to such an extent that it had become necessary to formulate new principles which would accommodate and predict possible health visiting experience. This led to the Education Committee of the C.E.T.H.V. setting up a Working Group in 1975.

1.2 Our terms of reference were to "examine the principles and practice of health visiting" as a pre-requisite to any major curriculum revision. We met for a total of seven half-day meetings and six week-ends. We were fortunate in not being given a time limit; and the way that we set about the task is, we believe, worthy of special comment. If a profession is to attempt to solve the problem of integration of theory and practice not only is a thorough re-appraisal of principles required, but it is also desirable to involve as many practitioners as possible. If the problem of relationship between theory and practice was to be solved, then in our opinion, these time-consuming activities were absolutely essential.

1.3 The health visitor tutors had expressed their concern, at the 1974 Wansfell Conference, that no further adaptations in the existing syllabus seemed possible and there was thus a need for a complete revision. We were, therefore, fully conscious of the need for changes to be made immediately; but if we had short circuited the stages of re-appraisal we would have satisfied only those who wanted immediate action. This in our opinion would not have provided a solution to the problem, but would in fact have intensified it, so creating further more urgent demands for changes in the near future. It was essential to provide feed-back as part of the participative process. This was done by circulating accounts of our on-going activities to members of the profession and this served to alleviate the anxieties of those wanting immediate solutions.

1.4 We learnt that the undertaking of a thorough re-appraisal meant that the solving of the problems created even more insecurity, particularly in the early stages. In the circumstances there was a temptation to contain the insecurity by involving as few people as possible in the revision. We decided however, that to bring about relevant change, the involvement of those demanding the change was necessary. Early in 1976 a workshop was held for health visitor tutors at Nottingham University, and this in turn led to the formation of local geographical groups, consisting of health visitors, fieldwork teachers, administrators and tutors. The findings from these groups were critically examined at a second workshop at Loughborough University held at the beginning of 1977. This time the participants reflected the membership of the local groups. (See Appendix 1.)

1.5 In order to formulate new principles it was necessary to have an agreed definition of health visiting. The following definition was agreed at our first workshop and accepted by most of the participants in the local groups.

"The professional practice of health visiting consists of planned activities aimed at the promotion of health and prevention of ill-health.

It thereby contributes substantially to individual and social well-being, by focusing attention at various times on either an individual, a social group or a community. It has three unique functions:

(1) Identifying and fulfilling self-declared and recognised as well as unacknowledged and unrecognised health needs of individuals and social groups.
(2) Providing a generalist health agent service in an era of increasing specialisation in the health care available to individuals and communities.
(3) Monitoring simultaneously the health needs and demands of individuals and communities; contributing to the fulfilment of these needs; and facilitating appropriate care and service by other professional health care groups."

1.6 An essential second phase was the clarification of concepts used in health visiting. The words used are often 'shorthand' and their original meanings have been forgotten. For example, we found the words used in some instances no longer conveyed the right meaning and new ones had to be found. In this context it was particularly helpful to have the assistance of Ruth Schröck, Lecturer, Edinburgh University. It was recognised that her uninhibited questioning of some fundamental assumptions underlying the practice of health visiting was necessary, since she did not share any of these assumptions. This made it impossible for us to seek refuge in established explanations since the concepts were meaningless unless the criteria for using them were spelt out in minute detail.

1.7 This led us to our main task which was to isolate the principles of health visiting. We took our original working definition of principles from 'Understanding Research in Nursing' by S. Chater (p.7). Here it was suggested that "principles state a relationship between two facts that may be used to explain, guide and predict action". It later became clear that there were other definitions, which have been used subsequently in this document. Principles should assist in teaching, evaluating and in providing an ideal model. Although we are fully aware of the difference in many instances between what is taught and what is or can be practised, we believe that the ideal provides a comparison for the ordering of reality, so as to achieve the best possible outcome.

1.8 The principles formulated are based on a belief in the value of health. If health, either as a measurable entity or as a subjective state of being, is of value and worthy of achievement then these principles must follow. Although listed sequentially, they are of equal importance in reflecting the process of health visiting.

(1) The search for health needs.
(2) The stimulation of the awareness of health needs.
(3) The influence on policies affecting health.
(4) The facilitation of health-enhancing activities.

A further discussion on the value of health and on each of the principles can be found in the following chapters.

1.9 From a set of accepted principles, it should be possible to derive the skills, attitudes and knowledge necessary to apply them in health visiting practice. The clarification of concepts should be an on-going process, otherwise there is the danger of stereotyping. As the concepts are redefined so there will be a need to reformulate the principles, but at some stage in the process of reappraisal conclusive statements must be made. Our intention has been to express the principles more scientifically, so that they can be subjected to rigorous evaluation.

Chapter 2

The Development of a Profession

The Changing Nature of Health Visiting
Activity in Relation to the Changes in
Conceptualization

2.1 The process of reappraisal necessitates a redefinition of concepts and this constituted one of the major activities of the Working Group in the early stages of its deliberations. The relationship which appears to exist between the concept of health and changes in society, politics, environment and technology over the past hundred years, and the evolution and the development of the profession constitutes a framework within which to review health visiting in its historical perspective.

Health Concepts in the Bacteriological Era
1840 to 1940

2.2 As Marie Collière says in her 'Thoughts on a New Approach to Public Health Nursing', the notion of health is relatively recent in the western world; it appears with the industrial era as a result of the new possibilities offered by the application of scientific discoveries. This was particularly so in the field of medicine, which in concentrating on bacteriological research could identify the causes of numerous illnesses which were both rampant and endemic. These discoveries considerably influenced the image of health which was considered for a comparatively long time as the absence of physical illness. Medicine had discovered the bacteria and germs which affect this or that organ, such as the pneumococcus, the meningococcus, Koch's bacillus, the tetanus bacillus. Thus to work for health meant to wage war against all these germs, to set up a whole plan of action, a complete strategic arsenal to drive back the lines of micro-biological aggression.[1]

Everything possible was done to fight against both health and social scourges, and to struggle to maintain life, particularly through all the activities undertaken to protect the mother and child. From this health concept arose the establishment of the basis of our health structures, and in particular the beginning of the personal health services of which health visiting is one. It is of interest to note, however, that the first health visitors were not nurses, and that their early activities were more akin to social work. The Voluntary Visiting Association under whose aegis they worked, had been formed in response to a crie de coeur from Thomas Turner (1793–1873) of the Manchester Royal Infirmary. He was concerned at the heavy loss of infant lives which was one of the evils resulting from the Industrial Revolution. He had first-hand experience of treating the marasmic dehydrated puny creatures who came to spend their last few hours in his ward, and he wanted visitors to go out to the homes from which these babies came and to seek out the causes of these wretched tragedies, which were due to mishandling by ignorant parents.[2]

The Nurse as a Health Visitor

2.3   Florence Nightingale (1820–1910) was amongst the first to point out the social aspects of infant mortality and to point the way to a practical remedy, by what she called household hygiene. In her notes on nursing (1858) she said "The same laws of health or of nursing, for they are in reality the same, obtain among the well as among the sick. The causes of the enormous child mortality are perfectly well known, they are chiefly want of cleanliness, want of ventilation, careless dieting and clothing, want of whitewashing; in one word defective household hygiene." Miss Nightingale felt that the work of "household hygiene" was a call to the nursing profession. At the age of seventy-one it occurred to her that the new local authorities (the County and County Borough Councils created in 1888) might be interested in this problem; she wrote to the chairman of the Technical Instruction Committee of her County. In this letter she said "it is hardly necessary to contrast sick nursing with this, (health visiting). The needs of home health bringing, require different but not lower qualifications and are more varied; they require tact and judgement unlimited to prevent the work being regarded as interference and becoming unpopular. She must create a new work and a new profession for women."[3] A special course of training was started and professional health visiting began (1892).

Education and Training

2.4   The early health visitors were selected rather than trained with emphasis on character, cleanliness and godliness. There was a missionary aspect to their work, and although medical discoveries in bacteriology were altering the ways in which illness was tackled, the notion of the miasmic theory of disease, (that theory which ascribed bad health to bad smells rather than to "bad" germs) continued to influence those who were fighting disease.[4] Later the emphasis was to be on the background of the worker; they could be doctors, sanitary inspectors, or nurses, and this choice no doubt was influenced by the growth of medical science and the need for the workers to be knowledgeable in this respect. However, the beginning, with its emphasis on day to day visits among the poor to teach and to help, was to be the corner stone of subsequent development. No generally recognised training existed for health visitors until 1919, when the new Ministry of Health and the Board of Education jointly promulgated a scheme for a two year course of training, normally to be associated with university institutions, which included training in social science and domestic subjects. However, trained nurses, graduates and women with three years' experience of health visiting might take a one year course; but at this time no midwifery qualification was required. In 1925 the Ministry of Health requested that in future midwifery training should be required for all health visitors. This development was understandable as maternal and child welfare services were being developed, and the implications of the Notification of Births Act (1915) were beginning to be felt in terms of continuity of service between midwife and health visitor. If families were to be visited following birth notification then visitors with some obstetric knowledge were necessary. However, this resulted in a reduction of training. The one year health visitor training was reduced to not less than six months, thus weakening the social and preventive preparation of the health visitor.[5] This concentrated attention on the maternal and child welfare aspects of the work, which gave necessary and immediate beneficial effects, held ultimate danger for the developing profession of health visiting. The two year course for health visiting was still an approved training, and with its emphasis on social and preventive care and on the principles of teaching, had undeniable advantages. However, it attracted fewer candidates, and an increasing number of local authorities showed preference for the health visitor who was already a trained nurse and midwife.

Statutory Qualifications

In 1929 the Local Government Act provided for statutory rules and orders setting out qualifications required for health visitors.

2.5 During the '30s the work of health visitors grew in importance as they and the doctors working in the public sector of the health service joined forces in the field of social medicine. This resulted in an expansion of training centres and an increase in the numbers of health visitors. The work was associated with the fall in infant and child deaths, and this association although helpful at the time (in that it was instrumental in diverting resources into training and employment), proved again to be somewhat of a two-edged sword. When war-time rationing and the introduction of welfare foods coupled with discoveries in the biochemical field dramatically reduced infant mortality, many people considered that the work of the health visitor had been completed. Recruitment declined and the number of training centres decreased from 32 in 1949 to 28 in 1954.[6] If the concept of health had not broadened at this time, it is conceivable that the health visitor as such might have disappeared.

The Welfare State

As it happened the concept of the welfare state with its insistence on the abolition of Beveridge's five giants, (disease, want, ignorance, squalor and idleness), saw a new and emerging role for the health visitor, which was enshrined in section 28 of the National Health Service Act 1946, the main tenets of which are further amplified in the subsequent section on legislation. It was some time before the effects of this new thinking were to be felt in terms of health visiting. However, the developing understanding of the relationship between the mental and social aspects of health and their implications for health visiting were beginning to be incorporated in the health visitor's work and training. In 1963 when the function of the health visitor was being re-defined for the purpose of redesigning the syllabus, knowledge of this relationship was almost, but not totally incorporated into the function. The C.E.T.H.V.'s leaflet on 'The Function of the Health Visitor' states, "the prevention of mental, physical and emotional ill-health is one of the five main aspects of the health visitor's work."[7] Social aspects of the work had been left out, but this might be explained by the need at that time to make a clear distinction between the role and function of the health visitor and the role and function of the social worker. This omission in the 'function' document does not signify that this important aspect has not been included before and after 1963, in both training and practice. It is implicit in the health visitor's work with families. However, the inclusion of the prevention of emotional disorder was a *new* factor so far as education and training were concerned. Dr. J. G. Howells in his paper to the C.E.T.H.V., at that time on the function and training of health visitors points out that although the health visitor's role is commonly defined as that of advisor and health educator on a variety of health and welfare problems, careful examination shows that many of these so-called 'welfare problems' are emotional in nature. Special training to increase the health visitor's awareness of this factor and the ability to manage and support families where such problems exist, was to be included in the new syllabus of training. Finally, it is important to show the limits of the W.H.O. definition of health, for even from the ideological point of view a state of complete well-being is not really compatible with life which is always effort and struggle.

Legislation and the Health Visitor

2.6 The results of local enquiries, reports and the achievements of science eventually find their way onto the statute books and are fed into the administrative machine of central and local government; there to be translated into nationwide measures for the protection of health. Health visiting has always been unusually sensitive to the effects of legislation, and very often Local Health Authorities and Local Education Authorities when fulfilling their duties and exercising their powers made use of health visitors. This has not always been in their best interests, nor that of the public. It is interesting to note that while on the one hand the 1946 National Health Service Act widened the scope of the health visitor's work adding care and after-care duties, which included giving advice as to the management of illness, including mental illness, on the other hand the Children Act of 1948 removed responsibility for certain aspects of child care from the health visiting service. Furthermore, at the very moment when this legislation was being implemented, the results of an investigation to determine how best to discover and identify the 'problem family',[8] showed that health visitors were the best and most reliable source of information, and that with suitable backing and training they should be able in the future to identify all such families in their areas. This pattern of reports and legislation which often contradict each other, and which are rarely properly implemented, together with the lack of clear role definition and the health visitor's occupational position on the boundaries of other work areas, led to anxiety caused on the one hand by the need for retraining for the new job, and on the other hand by a feeling that certain traditional areas of work were being encroached upon by other professional workers.

Education and Training in the 1950s and 1960s

2.7 In the 1950s, although the minimum period of training was still six months, an increasing number of courses extended the training to nine months. These courses were stimulated by an amended and broader syllabus which began in 1950 to prepare health visitors for their function envisaged in the National Health Service Act 1946. However, in spite of the expanded role and the extended training, recruitment to the service was poor. It became necessary to clarify the changed role of the health visitor and in 1953 a working party was set up to advise on the proper field of work, and on the recruitment and training of health visitors. The report, known as the Jameson Report[9], was published in June 1956. This important and only report on health visiting defined the function of the health visitor as primarily health education and social advice, but with the emphasis firmly on health education. Health visitors should continue, the report said, to keep contact with all families where there are children, but should be prepared to extend their role to become general family visitors. They had an important contribution to make in such fields as mental health, hospital after-care, and the care of the aged. They could provide a link to a wide variety of more specialised services and workers when required. The report recommended that registration as a nurse should continue to be a pre-requisite for training as a health visitor, but did not consider that the Part 1 Certificate of the Central Midwives Board provided suitable training, for future health visitors, in maternity care. It was, therefore, recommended that intending health visitors should either be state certified midwives, or have undergone a special three months' course in aspects of midwifery relevant to health visiting. Another main recommendation was that a new central training body should be set up representative of professional and educational interests and employing authorities, to devise a national syllabus, approve courses, and appoint examiners.

2.8 The Jameson Report was followed in due course by the Health Visiting and Social Work (Training) Act 1962, which set up the Council for the Training of Health Visitors, later to be named the Council for the Education and Training of Health Visitors, on the lines recommended in the report. One of the first tasks facing the Council on its inauguration in 1962 was the design of a new and comprehensive form of training to meet the needs of the health visiting service in the United Kingdom.[10] The plan of training which resulted, differed radically from the previous pattern. The Council had to take into account six main points:

(1) The wide variation in the deployment of public health nursing staff throughout the country, ranging from the triple duty nurse in rural areas undertaking health visiting along with domiciliary midwifery and district nursing, to the health visitor working in maternity and child welfare or the school health service, acting in liaison between hospital departments and the community, or specialising in particular problems such as those of the diabetic or the elderly. As distinct from this there was an increasing tendency to carry out health visiting within group medical practice where it was envisaged the range of duties would extend.

(2) The need to produce a syllabus flexible enough to allow for community changes and adaptation as the pattern of disease alters and the knowledge of their aetiology expands.

(3) The expanding knowledge gained from the sociological study of communities and their attitudes towards health.

(4) The growing appreciation of the significance of emotional factors in health and sickness.

(5) The changing demand on the service due to a better informed public which necessitates workers fully aware of their part in the community service and capable of explaining their role in the promotion of health and the prevention of disease.

(6) The advent in the health and welfare field of other workers capable of taking over some of the work the health visitor had had to carry in the past.[11]

The Aim of the Training

2.9 The pattern of training which came into operation in October 1965 was based on the view that the health visitor's task had two main aspects, firstly the assessment of the health potential of both the individual and the family group and provision of appropriate health education, and secondly, the assessment of the health needs of the handicapped of all age groups, the implication of their care for the family, and their continued maintenance and support in the community.[11] It was envisaged that the work could be carried out either in small geographically defined areas or by working within general medical practice. As already stated, health visitors in the early years of this century were not necessarily trained nurses. This was then changed and the new syllabus was based on a rule requiring candidates to be nurses on the general part of the state registers, with either a midwifery qualification or with approved experience in obstetric nursing. Candidates would therefore enter health visitor training with the knowledge of normal physiology and pathological processes, and considerable skill in observation, arising out of their period of work in hospital. This knowledge and this skill were to be expanded to fit them for community work. Consequently the syllabus was designed:

(a) to sharpen the student's capacity to perceive early deviations from the normal;

(b) to give knowledge of various statutory and voluntary agencies which may assist in any particular family situation;

(c) to provide practice in the working out of a programme of help for the individual where this is required;

(d) to prepare the student to select the method of health education likely to be the most successful in any particular instance.

To meet these aims the syllabus was divided into the following broad headings:

(1) Development of the Individual.
(2) The Individual in the Group.
(3) The Development of Social Policy.
(4) Social Aspects of Health and Disease.
(5) Principles and Practice of Health Visiting.

Principles and Practice

2.10 It is not possible in one short chapter to cover all aspects of the development of a profession and this perspective has touched on some but not all of the major influences which have shaped modern health visiting. A history of the first twelve years of the C.E.T.H.V. has already been commissioned, but a thorough examination of theoretical assumptions underlying health visiting practice has yet to be undertaken. It is clear however, that certain cherished beliefs about the education and training of health visitors have arisen since the inception of the C.E.T.H.V. and among these, has been the insistence on teaching underlying principles rather than current techniques so that the depth of understanding which allows an easy adaptation of basic knowledge to new problems and new conditions can be achieved. The profession has reached a stage where in order to develop further it must spell out the implicit principles which ultimately guide and predict its practice.

References

1. Collière, M. F. Thoughts on a New Approach to Public Health Nursing. Vol. 22, No. 6, p. 80. *International Nursing Review*. May/June 1975.
2. Brockington, F. C. *The Health of the Community*. p. 18. Churchill 1954.
3. Nightingale, F. Letters from Florence Nightingale on Health Visiting in Rural Districts.
4. Brockington, F. C. *The Health of the Community*. p. 18. Churchill 1954.
5. Hale *et al. The Principles and Practice of Health Visiting*. Pergamon Press 1968.
6. Ministry of Health, Department of Health, Scotland and Department of Education (1956). *An Enquiry into Health Visiting* (Jameson Report). H.M.S.O.
7. C.E.T.H.V. (1965). *The Function of the Health Visitor*.
8. Eugenics Society. An Investigation to determine how best to find out the existence of the problem family.
9. Ministry of Health, Department of Health Scotland and Department of Education (1956). An Enquiry into Health Visiting. (Jameson Report) H.M.S.O.

10. C.E.T.H.V. (1965). Syllabus Examination for Health Visitors in the United Kingdom.
11. C.E.T.H.V. (1965). Background to the Syllabus of Training.

Chapter 3

Health as a Value

3.1 What is health? Where does it begin and end? What does it mean to different people? There are many definitions which could be considered, but perhaps the most widely accepted is that of the WHO which describes health as a state of complete physical, mental and social well-being, rather than solely as an absence of disease.[1] Yet it is conceivable that this state can be achieved by some people who might otherwise be regarded as handicapped. This would be in agreement with Ruth Freeman's definition of health as a condition that maximises the individual's capacity to live happily and productively, that is the degree to which he is able to carry on his usual activities, or the level he can achieve, within the limits of pre-existing disease, disability or genetic endowment.[2] Professor Court and his Committee defined health by using a quotation from Katherine Mansfield "By health, I mean the power to live a full, adult, living breathing life in close contact with what I love—I want to be all that I am capable of becoming".[3]

3.2 Murray and Zeater have defined health as a purposeful, adaptive response, physically, mentally and socially, to internal and external stimuli, in order to maintain stability and comfort; and illness as a disturbed adaptive response, resulting in disequilibrium and inability to use the usual health promoting resources.[4] Since health itself is not viewed as absolute, the definition of 'health needs' follows an equally fluctuating pattern. Rine and Montag suggest they cover "those elements of living common to all human beings which are essential for functioning in organised society and which if not met lead to illness in body, mind or spirit".[5] Although these bio-phycho-social elements are primarily specific they become so interwoven as often to appear indistinguishable from one another.

3.3 If the state called 'health' is regarded as a continuum with the 'normal' being the point of balance between health and ill-health, the average person will rarely be at the same point for very long. In a survey undertaken in 1972 about nine out of ten people were shown to experience some symptoms of ill-health during the course of any two week period.[6] However, an individual is usually

20

regarded as officially healthy if he is not consulting his doctor; and even with elaborate diagnostic tests it has become difficult to define a total absence of disease. As Dubos indicates "Health is not a state of being . . . it is a process of adaptation to the changing demands of living and the changing meanings we give to life".[7] Ill-health may occur when there is a failure to respond to any of the changes of life. This means that when there is illness it is much more important to use *all* that remains of health, or to put it another way, to use the capabilities of life to contend with disease, rather than to concentrate on the disease itself.

3.4 Health can be seen as a state of being, but Katherine Mansfield and Dubos are suggesting that it is also important to consider it as the process of becoming, that is a movement from potentiality to actuality in all aspects of being, physical, emotional, social, intellectual and spiritual. Individuals interact with their environment on all of these planes and development from infancy onwards takes place by means of this interaction. Thus, there is not necessarily a unique state of being known as 'health', but a pattern of environmental responses which may lead an individual either away from, or towards, the achievement of his potential in any or all of the aspects of his being.

3.5 Value indicates worth, and as a concept involves value judgements. Thus recognition of a value can lead to the individual or the group achieving standards and accepting obligations of conduct. It may reflect what a person or society feels ought to be done, rather than what is actually done. A value should be based on adequate background knowledge and awareness of standards from which to make a choice. Knowledge produces a greater awareness of values, which in turn can influence behaviour. Acceptance of values does not necessarily mean that the ideas are adhered to, as social or personal pressures may militate against them, so their benefits may need to be reinforced by socially-acceptable sources.[8] All this is true of the value of health.

3.6 In an age of comparative affluence expectations in relation to many aspects of life are increasing—better living conditions, better wages and better health. Yet there is a danger in everyone expecting to be a paragon of health all the time, and the demand for medical care needs to be balanced by a greater awareness of personal responsibility for individual and community health. Perceptions and expectations of health will vary according to personal, cultural and ethnic background and patterns of work. The long-distance runner, the secretary, the ballet dancer will have different ideals of attainment. It may be necessary only to reinforce the individual's own methods of achieving optimum capacity, providing that these are within appropriate health norms; and consideration should be given to personal theories and beliefs. However, there must be an awareness of the dangers as well as benefits of dietary and other regimes which have periods of fashion or are of cultural origin, and which may be detrimental to health. The maintenance of good health for those who have it, the concern for those with impaired health, and the attaining of a better standard of health for others are principles of health visiting from which relevant theories may be deduced. Health visitors are concerned with the identification of the health needs of persons of any age group within the community, particularly those who are at potential risk of physical or mental breakdown. In this they are associated with other primary health care workers, although their role is predominantly in the field of promotion of health and prevention of disease.

3.7 One of the main functions of the primary health care team should be to promote, amongst the patients, a sound and practical attitude to healthiness, with the objective of creating a healthy population, which ultimately will not require its services. The primary health care team is concerned with the whole person and his lifestyle; and its most powerful ally is an educated public opinion. The main problems are the wide generality of the scope of the team and of the concept of health; and the difficulty of defining success. The public tends to get bored, in this, as in other spheres, with the less dramatic aspects of the subject. It needs to learn to appreciate the attractiveness of the positive value of health and how to use it to the full.[9]

3.8 It is the consumer who decides when he is sick and when to see a doctor. The latter may turn a minor ailment into an official illness by giving it a diagnostic label, which has a psychological effect upon the patient. The primary care team can help individuals through the health hazards of their life so that they are not encouraged to become invalids. While this may involve periodic medical treatment, there are many other factors concerned in the maintenance of health.[10]

3.9 Although there has been much improvement in the health of the nation over the past thirty years, due to a variety of developments including environmental factors, medical progress, and better educative services, particularly in the care of mothers and children, there is no room for complacency. There remain many areas where the environment has adverse effects on both the physical and mental health of people, be this by various types of pollution, methods of housing, noise or other causes. While we have cleansed our air by the development of smokeless zones many other problems remain, such as that of waste disposal. All workers in the health services could be more aware of the possibilities and opportunities to influence policies to improve health at the community level as well as at the individual level.

3.10 There are marked regional and class variations in the infant mortality rate, and in general morbidity, which are unacceptable if we wish to ensure that all children have an equal opportunity to enjoy good health. This is clearly emphasised by the Court Committee in its report "Fit for the Future".[11] These unacceptable differences in health care of children are also stressed in the Scottish Home and Health Department report "Towards an Integrated Child Health Service", which envisages the future need "to ensure that children reach adult life in the best physical, mental and emotional health that can be achieved".[12] It will be essential if these aims are to be achieved, to seek out and make more impact with those groups within the population which are not making adequate use of available health facilities.

3.11 Health visitors are unique in the health team because of their contact with the 'well' population and of their ability to visit families on their own initiative in the absence of crisis. This gives them an excellent opportunity for health education, both on a one-to-one basis in the home and in group situations. Prospective parents and those with young babies are usually at a particularly receptive period; and this is where a continuing relationship can be established with the family if there are enough health visitors to make it possible to undertake sufficient home visiting. The fall-off in clinic attendance and health surveillance after the age of one year which has been noted in many surveys, means that children are still reaching school age with undiagnosed defects. School children can have their interest captured in learning how their body works and more opportunity should be taken to link this with teaching on how to maintain health, and thus with the preparation of the parents of the future. The understanding and prevention of the various health crises of middle-age, the maintenance of health in the elderly, and the specific needs of ethnic groups are some of the many potential areas for health teaching by health visitors.

3.12 With better standards of obstetric and medical care, more mentally and physically handicapped people are surviving birth and childhood. It is vital to enable this group to achieve their potential and whenever possible to take part in the life of the community. The health visitor has an essential role in teaching, supporting, mobilising resources and liaising with other medical and caring professions to assist handicapped people and their families to achieve the best life possible for them.

3.13 One price of failing to teach positive attitudes towards responsibility for health, is the increasing use and immense cost of curative facilities. It is estimated that there is an increase in hospital admissions of $1\frac{1}{2}$–2% a year, in spite of the aim of the recent policies to care for more patients in the community.[13] The tax payer's money is paying for both prevention and cure, and it is difficult to demonstrate the economic benefits of prevention. It has been suggested that certain codes of good procedure and practice might be established which define tasks leading to an identifiable improvement in the service, and so aid evaluation. This was demonstrated by Dr. W. Ferguson Anderson and health visitors in Glasgow in relation to visiting the elderly.[14] Nevertheless, some preventive measures such as immunisation programmes have clearly resulted in a reduction in curative costs. Other programmes may yet need to be developed, for instance prenatal diagnosis for Downs Syndrome and spina-bifida. The cost of such programmes would be offset by fewer demands for long-term care, but their implementation would also involve active education in the need for early medical advice.

3.14 The number of working days lost through sickness is considerably greater than those lost by industrial disputes, and it is certain that some of this sickness is preventable. Chronic illness in professional classes is 5% as compared with 18% in unskilled manual workers, which has serious implications.[13] Although other factors than actual disease may be involved, it is agree that this is another area for prevention, and for further consideration of the illness behaviour of people who may report sick because of their uncertain value judgement as to what can be legitimately called illness. A more positive attitude towards health is needed, for frequently people are not interested in health maintenance nor in the behavioural changes which may be required to attain it.

3.15 The WHO definition of health is a three-dimensional concept and as discussed by Donald Hicks in 'Primary Health Care' it is extremely difficult to measure satisfactorily. It is suggested, however, that it should be possible to formulate a 'health status' index in addition to considering mortality, morbidity, and prevalence of illness, as is undertaken in the D.H.S.S. annual reports 'On the State of the Public Health'. One such index defines eleven states ranging between well-being and death, through mild symptoms and severe disability, which would cover the entire population; another suggests seven groups of states.[9] The development of any such project would involve a great deal of research, but it does illustrate the need to consider the state of the health of the population rather than only the ill-health. Could a health profile of the needs within a community division help to highlight the health status of a district?

3.16 More information could be given to the public, in easily assimilable and attractive form about the health statistics of their neighbourhood, so that there is a better understanding of immunisation states, improved mortality rates etc. In this way more interest can be aroused in promoting health standards.

3.17 The social value of health visiting activities can be wider than a combination of individual actions. Independent decisions may need to be co-ordinated to obtain an optimum use of resources, for the best maintenance of health at community and personal levels. To achieve these aims health visitors will need to have a sound knowledge of the essentials for good health, so that the work is founded on a scientific basis, and an understanding of research methods, so that investigations can be carried out to assess need. They will also need skills to enable them to communicate by appropriate and acceptable means, and an attitude of receptive awareness of indications of the health status of the individual and the community.

References

1. WHO (1948). Constitution.
2. Freeman, R. (1970). Community Health Nursing Practice. W. B. Saunders.
3. Mansfield, K. By permission of the Society of Authors.
4. Murray, R., Zeater, J. (1970). Nursing Concepts for Health Promotion. Prentice Hall.
5. Rine, A., Montag, M. L. (1976). Nursing Concepts and Nursing Care. Wiley Medical.
6. Dunnel, K. Cartwright A. Medicine Takers, Prescribers and Hoarders. Routledge & Kegan Paul.
7. Dubos, R. Mirage of Health. London Allen and Unwin 1960. Quoted in D. Hicks Primary Health Care Para. 138.
8. C.C.E.T.S.W. (1976). Values in Social Work. Paper 13, Chap. 2.
9. Hicks, D. (1976). Primary Health Care. Chapts. 1 and 2. H.M.S.O.
10. OHE (1975). The Health Care Dilemma.
11. DHSS (1976), Fit for the Future. Report of the Committee on Child Health Services. H.M.S.O.
12. Scottish Home and Health Department (1973). Towards an Integrated Child Health Service. Chapt. 2. H.M.S.O.
13. DHSS (1976). Prevention & Health, Everybody's Business. Chaps. III, IV and VII. H.M.S.O.
14. Anderson, W. Public Health Problems of an Ageing Population.

Chapter 4

The Search for Health Needs

4.1 If it is accepted that health is a value, and therefore an individual and community asset, it follows that searching for health needs and assisting in meeting them is a legitimate activity for health visitors, and this principle has been the most readily accepted. In this section we intend to examine the validity of 'search' as a principle of health visiting, and then to discuss some of its characteristics and implications.

4.2 Is search a principle? If by principle one means that search and its consequences are causally related, then the answer must be no. It cannot be claimed that because search occurs certain results can be predicted. At best it may be postulated that certain effects may recur occasionally. However, this is only one of four major definitions[1] of principle and two of the remaining three are applicable to 'search' in its health visiting context.

4.3 In the first place, historically, 'search' is a primary source, a primary element in health visiting. Our original employers sent health visitors into communities which had obvious and desperate health needs. It was left to the individual worker to search for and identify the health needs of individual families. Without this painstaking and time-consuming search the identification of individual need could not have been made with any precision, nor appropriate remedies applied. Within the framework of existing values and knowledge, and in co-operation with others, this tradition of the independent practitioner initiating her own search has been continuous and has been strengthened in health visiting. As health needs have become less overt search was, and is even more importantly now, the source of all health visiting practice.

4.4 Secondly, search is a fundamental truth of health visiting from which its reasoning stems. One cannot assess and treat until one has found and identified. There is a linear progression in reasoning (search, → identify, → assess,) however much the stages may be telescoped, or appear to happen simultaneously.

4.5 Using the definition of a principle as an origin, a primary element, and as a fundamental truth, then the search for health needs can be advanced as a principle of health visiting, for scrutiny by the profession. It is interesting that its acceptance has been unanimous so far by the members of the geographical working groups and of the workshops at Nottingham and Loughborough. There appears to have been an acknowledgement of something so fundamental to health visiting as to be unarguable, so obviously implicit that its explication is seen as a statement of the obvious.

4.6 Some of the workshop participants initially expressed disquiet about the term used, in that the word 'search' in normal use has connotations of inquisition, suspicion, aggression. Alternatives were suggested such as 'identification' or 'recognition'. The search for health needs would then read 'the identification or recognition of health needs'. However, both these words seem to lack the essential characteristics of the activity, that is the active deliberate looking initiated by the health visitor. The term 'search' implies an intention to find, whereas 'identification' and 'recognition' suggest something already found[2]. The discussion over the word does suggest that we may be at the stage of needing to develop more specific terminology in order to be more precise both to ourselves and to others about what we do.

4.7 In the context of health visiting 'search' is regarded as an activity that is purposeful, unique, focused on health, self initiated, expert and non-stigmatising. The quality of the search is constrained by overriding ethics and client participation. Some of these aspects of the activity are considered in detail in the following paragraphs.

4.8 The purpose of the search is to look for acknowledged and un-acknowledged health needs. Its basic premises are that health is desirable, and attainable; and that it is definable to such an extent that factors promoting good health as well as signs and symptoms of ill-health can be isolated and identified. It follows then that it is possible for health needs to be identified.

There are obvious problems in making this identification. Within a society or between individuals there will be conflicting definitions both of health needs and of their ranking in order of importance. Since health itself is not viewed as absolute, the definition of health needs must follow an equally fluctuating pattern. Whilst there may be agreement on physiological needs, perception of other health needs is relative. In particular health needs identified by the individual or family may not be similarly perceived by the health visitor and vice versa. Bradshaw has an approach to 'need definition' which is discussed later in this document. Moreover whilst absolute (physiological) needs are probably immutable, relative needs will change as the pattern of disease, and of expectations of health and health services, change[3].

4.9 Even given that there could be agreement on the identification of existing health needs the health visitor is in a position to identify emerging problems as needs, before there is general awareness, 'expert' agreement or societal willingness to admit the need. This has educational implications. The student needs knowledge, not only of accepted health needs, but also of the criteria used for identifying them, including the ability to evaluate those criteria.

4.10 However, in spite of the problems of identifying health needs, in practice health visitors are aware of those that are generally known and agreed and are able to identify them in individuals, families and the community. Primarily, there is a health need when a want of health can be foreseen. As a consequence of present behaviour and/or of environmental factors it is possible to predict likely outcomes for individual, family and community health (eg. smoking; inconstant inadequate child-rearing patterns; excess noise). A health need exists when a want of health can be foreseen as a result of future human development about which individuals may lack knowledge (eg. parental education while their child is a baby to ensure a safe environment for him when he becomes a toddler; pre-retirement education). Secondarily, a health need is present when health is absent i.e. illness. Any needs may be acknowledged or unacknowledged, recognised or not recognised. If the latter, this may be due to lack of knowledge, lack of insight, or because of emotional barriers.

4.11 The search for health needs is purposeful because health visitors know what they are looking for, as well as how to search (see below) and why (see Chapter 3—Health as a Value).

4.12 The search for health needs by the health visitor is unique. Health visiting is the only profession whose primary aim is to promote personal health by searching for health needs and helping individuals, families and groups to provide for them. Moreover, its original raison d'être has been confirmed and recognised as it has developed. The distinct task of deliberately seeking out health needs has been a feature of health visiting since its inception[4] and is mentioned also in recent publications such as that of Thurmott.[5] Some members of other professions also look for unreferred personal health needs—for instance community physicians and occupational health staffs.

4.13 Also unique is the major setting for the identification of health needs. This setting can include the home, the clinic, the surgery and school and, since

1968,[6] the hospital. However, the emphatic confirmation of the home as the paramount setting was marked in the thinking of the geographical groups, and those health visitors at Nottingham and Loughborough. There is no other occupational group in the health or social services with the tradition of visiting people in their own homes, so that health needs may be identified before health problems develop.

4.14 To the same end moreover this visiting occurs at times of non-crisis as well as crisis. The visits may be initiated by the health visitor; by the person visited; or may result from referral. Both non-crisis visiting and its routine initiation by the health visitor are unique.

4.15 Stated in this way the obvious questions become apparent. Is this a description of the reality of practice?[7] If not, why not? Is the only reason resource constraints? To what degree do environmental and social conditions and the provision of complementary or auxiliary services affect the possibility of applying the search principle i.e. practising health visiting? What administrative settings facilitate or hinder the search for health needs? What kind of education best equips practitioners?

4.16 The nature of the search is expert, and this implies that the search has a known aim, adequate methods, adequate resources and is professional and based upon knowledge. It has been suggested already that the health visitor knows pragmatically what health needs are, however difficult it is in theory to define both health and health needs. Given an awareness of these difficulties and a respect for them, it is perfectly feasible that a health visitor can make a first visit, say to a family with a new baby, and know immediately what possible health needs that family may have. The search is purposeful and informed before the health visitor has met the family or knows anything about them. Time is needed to search, identify, recognise and assess the specific health needs of that particular family. Time is needed both for observation and for the establishment of a relationship through which needs can be recognised and the subsequent stages, relative to this and other principles, be carried through. Obviously in practice some or all of the principles in health visiting are being applied simultaneously. In the sense that they are practised, skilled and knowledgeable health visitors are conducting an aimed expert search.

4.17 During times of economic stringency constraints may be placed on the active searching out process on the grounds that some work must be left undone to enable crisis work to be undertaken. It is notoriously difficult to prove the economic worth of prevention, especially when it can be justifiably argued that raising public awareness of health needs may increase demands on hard pressed services.[8] Equally it can be argued that early detection and prompt referral of need may result in less expenditure in the long term. Clearly there are many contradictory issues here. Rising consumer expectations may mean the constant presentation of new needs. Needs may be highlighted which the community itself might suggest meeting by alternative and possibly innovatory ways. Constraints upon searching by the health visiting service may also arise because of the inability of other services to fulfil their own special obligations in meeting needs.

4.18   The expert nature of the search is apparent in the method used which consists of observation, interpretation and deductions from data. Validation by collecting new facts to refute or confirm the hypothesis, follows. In reality this is generally the weak link in the practice of health visiting, as we all know, and this was particularly emphasized at Loughborough. It is, therefore, imperative to devise tools of evaluation in health visiting.

4.19   There are problems if one assumes that the scientific method is the most desirable or the only method which can be used by health visitors to search. For various reasons it is difficult to apply the scientific method in full to human beings. This way of looking at reality involves making assumptions about the nature of human beings as rational individuals and about the possibility that values can be inferred from behaviour. It is suggested that there is another dimension in addition to the scientific in the health visitor's methods of search, but further thinking and research will be needed to make this explicit.

4.20   Without the participation of the client only the most overt needs can be observed and that to no further purpose. The extent to which any worker can explore the health state of an individual or a group, and the environmental or personal factors affecting this, will be tempered by the degree to which the clients are willing to respond and co-operate. Although legislation confers a responsibility on the Health Authority to provide a health visiting service which offers advice on health needs, the health visitor quite rightly has not statutory right of entry to homes; and furthermore no one is obliged to use the service. Hence the profession itself has to constantly re-appraise the limits and form of its intervention.

4.21   Inherent in the health visiting search process is the recognition of the uniqueness and worth of individuals, their right to receive respect and their right to freedom and dignity. Any seeking out of needs must, therefore, be a participative process, undertaken within the framework of the personal philosophy and cultural value systems of the client, and with self-determination accorded the client, as far as is compatible with the rights and needs of others. Individuals and groups often cling to deeply entrenched habits and may resist efforts to change them. Individuals vary in their awareness of, and willingness to acknowledge, needs so it is clearly important that each client is made aware of the role and function of the health visitor and the intention of the search process. The integrity as well as the skill of the worker is reflected in the way in which the service is presented and in the manner in which the client's health behaviour is observed.

4.22 Having examined the characteristics of search and discussed some of the implications, certain conditions necessary for successful search have become clear. There are certain pre-requisites if the search for health needs is to be successful, and some of these have been referred to already. However, it might be helpful to collate them before discussing them further and considering some of their implications.

Essential factors for successful search are:

(1) The initiation and development of a relationship such that any needs will become apparent and may be acknowledged. In most cases this requires contact (probably by routine home visiting) over a period, so that normal health, deviations from it and potential health needs can be identified.
(2) The motivation and ability to initiate the search.
(3) Knowledge.
(4) Skills.

4.23 The establishment of the relationship requires commitment, communication skills, and time. Probably the greatest single constraint on effective search is the acknowledged shortage of health visitors, as well as the transience of health visitors in certain areas.[9] Given the need to spend time on establishing a relationship, but knowing that time may not be or is not available, it becomes important to develop that pattern of visiting which is most likely to give high returns. Less random and more effective health visiting could be practised by visiting at known critical points in the life-cycle. Health visitors have always recognised 'critical periods' for identifying certain health needs, such as during the ante or post natal period, at certain points of child development and at other periods of adult development. Also there are those episodes in life that are known to produce health needs, for example moving to a new area, bereavement, illnesses. It may be argued that people are more likely to be receptive of health help when their health needs are more apparent.

4.24 If the view is taken that searching will be most effective if undertaken at these specific stages of development or at times of physiological or psycho-social stress, then the aggregation of these 'critical periods' for a given population might serve as the basis for quantitatively estimating the minimum number of visits needed for effective search and health promotion in that population. (Of course any such attempt to assess health needs and therefore the number of health visitors required would have to take account of other factors judged relevant to health e.g. environmental and social conditions, family size, family employment and income etc.). However, just as the concept of selective screening has fallen into disrepute because it proved impossible to ensure the normality of the excluded 'normal' group, so the concept of vulnerable periods in the life span has yet to be tested rigorously.

4.25 If health visitor students need to acquire knowledge about techniques and methods of data analysis, they will require education in logical, critical thinking and in scientific method. A questioning attitude and the ability to evaluate and apply research findings is necessary. Data collection and history taking will need to be undertaken more systematically and this will require greater attention to be paid to record keeping and, probably, to the standardisation of records so that information may be retrieved and compared more readily. Skills in observation, listening and communicating are also needed[10] and this implies deepening knowledge of the behavioural sciences and the strengthening of the practitioner skills of counselling and enabling. Attitudes and traits appropriate to the tasks of identifying and highlighting health needs and securing their recognition will require deeper exploration, and the use of material from ethics, philosophy and political science. Because cultural factors within a pluralistic society increasingly affect health, epidemiological and sociological knowledge will also need to be deepened. Students are likely to be better equipped to search effectively if educational methods encourage in them an ability to find information rather than to rely on memory; demand thought rather than habitual modes of behaviour; and encourage a questioning attitude rather than a passive acceptance.

4.26 In conclusion, it is suggested that the search for health needs is indeed fundamental to health visiting and is in fact a principle of health visiting. The problems associated with it lie in the education of students, as well as in the application of this principle to practice in a period of continuing scarcity of resources.

References

1. The Shorter Oxford Dictionary.
2. Discussed by R. Shrock at Loughborough.

3. Lewis, A. (1953). Health as a Social Concept. B.J.S.4.109. Susser, M. & Watson, W. (1962). Sociology in Medicine O.U.P. Titmus, R. (1958). Essays on the Welfare State. Allen & Unwin. Leighton, A. & Murphy, J. (1965). The Problem of Cultural Distortion. Millbank Memorial Fund Quarterly. 2.189.
4. Nightingale, F. (1891). Letter to F. Verney. Clark, J. (1973). A Family Visitor R.C.N.
5. Thurmott (1976). Health and the School. R.C.N.
6. Public Health Service Act. (1968).
7. Laker, K. Adjusting to being a Health Visitor. Nursing Times, 30.9.76.
8. Radical Statistics Health Group, Whose Priorities? p. 16.
9. DHSS (1976). Report of the Committee on Child Health Services (Court). Vol. II, Tables F12, F13; Regional and Area Profiles G.1. Vol. I. 6.19 p. 97.
10. Freeman, R. (1973). Community Nursing Practice.

Chapter 5

Stimulation of an Awareness of Health Needs

5.1 In the previous chapters discussion has centred on health as a value and the search for health needs. In this chapter the emphasis will be on the stimulation of an awareness of health needs and the engendering within the individual and the community of personal responsibility for meeting these needs. In attempting to clarify health needs, both the concepts of 'health' and of 'needs' should be examined more closely.

5.2 The WHO definition of health discussed in a previous chapter aims to achieve a very high ideal and it is worth while giving the statement emphasis because so often health is only considered in a neutral or even negative way, whilst for the health visitor it indicates a goal of positive well-being. It is however, for many of our clients, an impossible goal to achieve. Another definition, by Freeman, is "the degree to which the individual is able to carry on his usual activities or the level the individual can achieve within the limits of pre-existing disease disability or genetic endowment"[1] This is perhaps more realistic and attainable, particularly if one is discussing the health needs of the handicapped and the elderly.

5.3 'Need' in the Oxford Dictionary is defined as want, requirement, necessity or state that requires relief. Bradshaw[2] has an approach based on the following definitions:
   (a) Normative need: this is what the experts, administrators or professionals define as need in any given situation.
   (b) Felt need: this is need equated with want.
   (c) Expressed need: this is felt need translated into action.
   (d) Comparative need: this is a measure of need found by studying the characteristics of those who are receiving a service and comparing them with people of similar circumstances who are not receiving a service.

34

Need may also be relative or anticipated. A further qualifying dimension of need is given by M. H. Cooper in 'Rationing Health Care' when he writes that "need can also be a matter of fashion".[3]

5.4 In 'Prevention and Health: Everybody's Business',[4] the four main groups of health problems facing society to-day are discussed, and in considering these groups certain health needs emerge, viz—those associated with an ageing population, with environmental and social conditions, with adverse life-styles, and with mental health needs.

5.5 Health needs associated with an ageing population.

During the last two decades major changes within the structure of the population have occurred. The over 65 population has increased by 25% and the over 75 age group is expected to rise by 500,000 over the next ten years from 2,300,000 to 2,800,000. Approximately 95% of elderly people live in their own homes, the remaining 5% are the heaviest users of health and personal social services.[5] The health needs of the elderly are increasing as the proportion in the population continues to rise, resulting in an ever rising demand for health care.

Anderson[6] considers prevention of illness is the most important aspect of future work in the management of elderly people and suggests there are three lines of approach to health care for this section of the population:

(i) Preserving as far as possible the physical health of the individual as age advances.
(ii) The maintenance of mental health.
(iii) Preservation of the social standing and circumstances of older people.[6]

5.6 Health needs associated with environmental and social conditions. The provision of an environment that is free of dangerous hazards has for many years been the aim of the health visitor and of the community occupational health services. Accident prevention in the community and in the home presents a major health need. If all drivers and front seat passengers wore seat belts 14,000 serious and fatal injuries would be averted, and £50,000,000 of expenditure saved every year; but even more deaths occur as a result of home accidents than because of road accidents.[7]

Environmental pollution presents a further major health hazard and dissemination of knowledge on the risks of chemical poisoning, eg. from pesticides, is again a growing health need. The environment is only partly physical, and the isolation of families in high-rise flats may give rise to mental trauma equally as disastrous to health as any chemical pollution which is also, in the long term, less easy to remedy. Teaching and helping young mothers to provide and maintain a stimulating but safe environment is a task of the health visitor.

Equally disadvantageous to children and their families is the deprivation suffered from living in the decaying, declining inner areas of our large cities. To encourage and stimulate an awareness of health needs, to motivate individuals and families to improve their own conditions, to take community action for better housing, schools, play areas and health services by teaching the value of health, must be a priority of health visitors and others.

Over the past 30 years, there has been a steady improvement in child health. There is still, however, very little room for complacency when the marked regional and social class variations are studied as is clearly evident in the Court Report 'Fit for the Future'.[8]

The recent report on neonatal and infant mortality issued in February 1977 by the Wirral Area Health Authority, further highlights this social class distinction.[9]

	Infant Mortality Rate		Perinatal Mortality Rate
	Legitimate	*Illegitimate*	
Birkenhead & Wallasey Primarily Social Class IV & V	20	38	27
Remainder of Wirral Primarily Social Class II and III	12	—	17
England and Wales	15	22	19

Owen shows that preventive health statistics emphasise existing inequalities, (e.g., variation in infant mortality rates in different regions, variations in death rates between social classes, regions and groups, marked morbidity differences between occupations) and suggests that analysis of the reasons why these differences exist would be beneficial. He cites factors that may explain the different health records between countries, regions, and groups e.g., heredity, climate, environment, life style, diet, exercise, smoking, alcohol, work satisfaction, the kind of health and social services provided and their cost, the use made of them, education and income.[10]

Certain of these factors may be altered or controlled. Pre-natal diagnosis (amniocentesis) cannot guarantee the development of a normal child, but it may prevent the birth of a grossly affected individual if abortion takes place. Further developments in testing maternal blood serum may enable highly selective amniocentesis to be carried out, reducing further the already small risk of aborting a normal foetus.[11]

The Sheffield Study on Sudden Infant Deaths has shown the effective contribution, in an area of previously unmet need, which can be made by an adequate number of health visiting staff co-ordinated so as to concentrate on a specific group. This type of work involves all aspects of the health visiting functions outlined in the Function of the Health Visitor (C.E.T.H.V.).[12]

5.7 Health needs associated with adverse life styles.

While the affluence consequent upon industrialisation has increased life expectancy for high proportions of populations, it has also contributed to over-indulgence in the use of food, alcohol and drugs. Technological developments in transport and communication have reduced the need for human physical activities which, combined with the stresses of competitive urban living, has led to a high incidence of cardio-vascular diseases. Environmental pollution created by industries and addiction to cigarette smoking increase the incidence of bronchial diseases and lung cancers.

The borderlines between health and sickness have become blurred. Obesity, alcoholism, depression, bereavement, sexual deviations and strained family relationships are increasingly being regarded as diseases justifying medical treatment. These sorts of social and mental disorders were previously regarded as problems for the individual, his family or perhaps the police courts or the church. Now, the health services are expected to take some responsibility for them thus producing a dependence on health personnel for help in coping with problems of living. Because of this the public have unlimited scope for regarding themselves as ill and for seeking medical solutions to their problems. It has been said that "a healthy person is, nowadays, one who has not been examined".[13]

"The current health problems discussed are mainly self-induced by individuals' ways of life or related to the inevitable degeneration accompanying the ageing process. Attempts by health professionals to 'cure' these conditions transform people into 'patients' producing passivity and the removal of self-responsibility for the resolution of their problems which is inherent in the process of being defined as ill".[14]

"To overcome the problems of obesity, addiction to alcohol, drugs or cigarettes, to change a stressful way of life or to adjust to bereavement requires the motivation and active particpation of those who have such difficulties if changes are to be created in their lives".[15] Often the solutions presented involve the use of drugs, but it is now being suggested that, far from providing help in resolving problems, the widespread use of drugs can reduce an individual's ability to develop self-coping mechanisms and may in fact lower levels of health.[16] For example, expenditure by the public in 1973 on alcohol and tobacco amounted to 15% of total consumer expenditure. In the same year 50,000 people died from smoking-related conditions, 2,000 people died of cirrhosis of the liver or alcohol poisoning and 500,000 people suffered the problems of alcoholism.[17]

5.8 Health needs associated with mental health.

The relationship between age, environment, life style and mental health is complex and time will not allow a detailed study of their influence on well-being. Equally it will not allow a study of the anxiety and depression which characterises the great majority of cases of diagnosed mental illness.

Between the years 1955–56 and 1970–71 the number of consultations with G.P.s in relation to mental illness doubled, with the diagnosis of neurotic depression increasing over twenty times; an estimated 5,000,000 patients attend for such consultations each year. Accurate interpretation of these figures is difficult as possible changes in the classification of disease have occurred, eg. a 50% fall in diagnosis of menopausal symptoms. In addition, whilst statistics show a falling rate of suicide they also demonstrate a steadily increasing number of people attempting suicide by self poisoning.

With some 600,000 mentally ill patients receiving specialist psychiatric care each year,[18] the prevention of mental illness by health teaching on psycho-social needs from infancy, should be one of the health visitor's main priorities. To stimulate awareness of health needs is a function of the health visitor, which is shared by others in the medical, educational and social fields. One of the objectives of primary health care is to encourage a positive and practical approach to health. For this to be possible a well informed public opinion is necessary. This may be achieved by a variety of health education measures, ranging from the use of mass media on a national or local scale, through the provision of special health programmes based in clinics, health centres and schools, to health teaching on a one to one personal basis.

5.9 It is a matter of regret that the media is not always positive in its presentation of health topics and often dramatises emotive sickness-orientated situations. The caring professions may not be aware of or prepared in advance for this, and are then often at a great disadvantage in dealing with the resultant problems, eg. recent infant feeding and immunization controversies. Increased consumer demands which are not conducive to positive health may also be stimulated by the media. For instance, the demand for sweets may be increased while the effects of dental caries are ignored.

5.10 The ways in which health visitors may attempt to stimulate awareness of health needs begin with their unique function in visiting all families. On their visits they will be able to assess the needs of the individual or family and on-going health teaching will take place. This specific teaching assessed in relation to personal health needs will enable information, relevant to the particular situation, to be given and may provide the basis from which responsible decisions can be made.

5.11 Health education on a micro level will hopefully result in a greater awareness in the community of specific needs and so encourage community action and in the long term possibly bring about changes in local or national health policies. Clearly, to stimulate awareness of health needs is an activity in which the client and the health visitor must jointly participate, with a recognition by the health visitor of the need for the individual to take decisions to deal with his own health and life situation.

5.12 These decisions will depend on the experience and health values of the client, which are not constant. Values change in relation to such factors as age, financial and health states and the current health and social norms of the individual in the community. To work together effectively, the recipient of advice and care must feel that the health visitor's primary objective is the good of the family. There must be mutual confidence. Health visitors must accept the existence of motivations that result in behaviour patterns different from those that they themselves would consider the norm.

5.13 Implementation of this principle may be difficult because of needs being perceived differently by the client and the health visitor. Situations may arise where the unconsciously or consciously held health values of the client and the health visitor may be in conflict due to differing social backgrounds, culture patterns and health values. However where there is mutual trust, built on a continuing relationship, it is possible for productive inter-action to take place.

5.14 The client may reject the advice or health teaching offered because of these unconsciously held values, or the rejection may be made on an informed basis, following free two-way communication. On the other hand, the client may decide that the teaching is relevant and alter his life style or modify some part of it, to a more positive health behaviour pattern. Health visitors provide information and anticipatory guidance and clients have the freedom to make their own decisions as to whether they should accept the information and advice or not.

5.15 "The health visitor characteristically operates in the wide area which lies between the mere provision of information on the one side and the use of legal compulsion on the other. Between these two is the area of the individual's right to act only under his own full and free consent, the health visitor mediating to him the judgement of the community (at its most informed and wisest) on how that consent should be exercised. 'Human beings owe to each other help to distinguish the better from the worse and encouragement to choose the former and avoid the latter. They should be for ever stimulating each other to . . . increased direction of their feelings and aims towards the wise instead of foolish".[19]

5.16 A question is again raised as to the desirability of stimulating an individual's awareness of need which cannot effectively be met, arousing undue anxiety about health. At the same time, a desirable level of self-help activity may be started. It may follow that aspects of need which cannot be dealt with immediately might well be fulfilled in the longer term, once they are uncovered and recognised; for example, where no nursery education is available the health visitor could co-operate with parents in establishing play groups.

In the past it may not have been a deliberate feature of health visiting practice to engage in participative activity with the community but a new partnership approach will be needed.

5.17 As has already been said, it is notoriously difficult to prove the economic worth of prevention and it can be argued that raising public awareness of health needs may simply increase the requests for additional health provisions. However, as previously discussed, there is growing evidence to show that public demand and medical responses may sometimes lead to over-reaction in respect of conditions which are more psycho-social than medical, resulting in increasing expenditure on services. It is pertinent to examine the stimulation of health needs at the level of primary and secondary prevention, especially when they may be dealt with by less costly and more effective techniques, such as self-help. An intensive care unit is more dramatic in its appeal than routine screening, but the latter serves many more people with much less expenditure. The public need to learn more about the advantages of the positive values of health and how to use them to the full, and less about sickness-orientated problems. This necessitates a major change in attitudes towards health throughout the population—a change in the

Number of Practising Health Staff in Great Britain

Registered Nurses	76,856	(whole-time equivalent)
Hospital Medical Staff	31,473	(whole-time equivalent)
State Certified Midwives	15,186	(whole-time equivalent)
General Practitioners	25,849	(absolute number)
District Nurses	12,793	(whole-time equivalent)
Health Visitors	8,240	(whole-time equivalent)

Number of Practising Health Staff per 100,000 Population

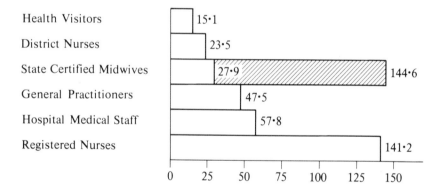

Notes

1. Statistics taken from D.H.S.S. 'Health and personal social services statistics for England with summary tables for Great Britain, 1975'. Population of Great Britain taken as 54,422,000.

2. The number of state certified midwives, of whom 10,799 are hospital based, and 4,387 community based, is 144·6 to every 100,000 females of a child-bearing age (i.e. 15–44 years). See shaded area in diagram. The number of females aged 15–44 is taken as 10,499,000.

philosophical thinking of government, in policies, priorities and in resource allocation. The projected cost of the National Health Service for the year ending March 1976 was approximately £5,000 million and at the same time, the projected health education expenditure amounted to less than 1% of the total N.H.S. Budget.[20]

5.18 The health needs that exist within the community have been discussed together with the health visitor's function. One point that has not been discussed is the very real fear of the profession that it will not be possible to carry out this task, due to the inadequate provision of resources. The health visiting profession has a responsibility for the health of the whole population. This claim is idealistic at a time when the number of health visitors is in such a poor proportion to the population as illustrated by the accompanying figures. With the reduction, or lack of increase, in other staff, especially in inner urban areas, health visitors in the 1970s have found themselves responding to crisis situations. In despair about their staffing problems, some have said that normal routine visits of health visitors are a luxury that cannot be afforded. This enforced change of role for health visitors is to be resisted, as once lost, it will be extremely difficult to recover this unique sphere of operation. Their visiting indeed must be planned, but, as was said earlier, not in response to crisis, but precrisis, and at such times as they, with their knowledge, know that a visit may be useful to a particular family.

5.19 Objectives have to be clearly defined and broken down into their basic elements before individuals, groups and communities can understand their own and others' health needs and with insight take responsibility for meeting them. Whether in relation to governments, or to individuals, awareness of health needs may not in itself be sufficient for the achievement of health. At this juncture it may be useful to consider the principle of 'influence'.

References

1. Freeman, R. (1970). Community Health Nurse. Chap. 1, p. 4. W.B. Saunders Co.
2. Bradshaw, J. (1972). A Taxonomy of Social Needs. p. 69. Oxford Univer. Press for Nuffield Provincial Hospitals Trust.
3. Cooper, M. H. (1975). Rationing Health Care. Chap. III, p. 21. Croom Helm, London.
4. DHSS (1976). Prevention and Health: Everybody's Business. Chap. VIII, p. 91. HMSO.
5. Owen, Dr. D. (1976). In Sickness and in Health, Chap. II, p. 29. Quartet Books London.
6. Anderson, W. F. (1976). Practical Management of the Elderly. Chap. III, p. 37. Blackwell Scientific Publications.

7. Owen, Dr. D. (1976). In Sickness and in Health. Chap. 10, p. 121, Quartet Books London.
8. DHSS (1976). Fit for the Future. Report of the Committee on Child Health Services. HMSO.
9. Wirrall Area Health Authority (1977). Report on Neonatal and Infant Mortality.
10. Owen, Dr. D. (1976). In Sickness and in Health. Chap. 10, p. 171. Quartet Books London.
11. DHSS. (1976). Prevention and Health, Everybody's Business. Chap. VI. HMSO.
12. Emery, J. et al. Unexpected death in infancy. Child Development Team, Sheffield.
13. OHE (1971). Prospects in Health.
14. OHE (1971). Health Care Dilemma, p. 7.
15. Swayne, J. (1976). Medicine and healing—a broken marriage. New Society.
16. Pills won't solve your problems. Brewer Collins.
17. OHE (1975). Medicines which affect the mind, p. 35 and p. 26.
18. DHSS (1976). Priorities for Health and Personal Social Services in England. Chap. VIII, p. 54. HMSO.
19. Baker, E. Is there a case for re-defining the role of the health visitor?—including quote from J. S. Mill on Liberty Chap. 4. Unpublished paper.
20. DHSS (1976). Priorities for Health and Personal Social Services in England, p. 82. HMSO.

Chapter 6

The Influence on Policies
Affecting Health

6.1 Implicit in the heading to this chapter is the principle that health visitors seek to influence policies affecting health and from this it follows that if successful there will be an outcome, that is, people's health will be affected in some way. If it is accepted that health is of value and worthy of achievement, then the health visiting profession has a responsibility to influence policies that affect health and in order to achieve this, health visitors will have to engage in political activity. To many people these statements will be disturbing because of the interpretation they may put on words such as 'influence' and 'politics' for these words are seen by some as meaning 'being obstructive', 'seizing power', or 'being revolutionary'.

6.2 In discussions held with members of the profession so far there was general agreement with the principle, but some concern over the wording unless it was defined and qualified. In scanning the literature relevant to the concepts of professional influence and political activity, there was a great deal of evidence to support the principle, but the words 'influence', 'policies', and 'politics' although used freely, were used in the main without definition, but always in the sense of being constructive. By 'influence' is meant 'to have an effect upon' or 'to be listened to' and it is not used in the sense of being obstructive or revolutionary. A 'policy' is interpreted as a course of action, procedure or strategy, determined informally by small groups or formally by local or national governments or authorities.

6.3 According to M. Duverger,[1] politics can be defined as the science of organised power in all communities and Dr. D. Owen,[2] when discussing the role of Community Health Councils considers that in a democracy access to information is power. Because the health visitor has relevant knowledge, skills and experience and has access to information, he or she has a responsibility as a professional person to influence policies that could affect people's health.

44

6.4 In everyday parlance to behave politically is often intended and construed to mean to be involved in interaction between individuals or within small groups in which the actions of one person are influenced by the actions of another, that is, a particular form of social behaviour is implied. Courses of action relevant to people's health are planned and carried out by all manner of organisations and individuals ranging from private industrial companies and voluntary organisations to individuals in related professions. In other words, a course of action relevant to someone's health could conceivably be planned and carried out by anyone. The difference between political behaviour associated with government, and what is in essence another and different type of social behaviour, is discussed by D. Raphael[3] who suggests that the word 'political' is robbed of its special meaning pertaining to government if it is used in the other sense to incorporate social behaviour between individuals or within small groups, although as he says not all political scientists would agree with him. Raphael also uses the word 'influence' in connection with pressure groups and politicians; and because the profession can exert influence by being a pressure group, this term must be defined since it is open to misinterpretation. The term is well discussed in the Open University unit on Health.[4] Pressure groups are taken to be those organised groups of people who seek to influence the decisions of Government without seeking at the same time, to become the Government. The section goes on to say that the action or inaction of Government often impels professional groups to act as pressure groups. An example is given of the medical profession which rarely had to act in this way before the state contemplated some measure of intervention in the provision or regulation of medical care.

6.5 In order to examine the implications inherent in the principle it is necessary to consider the nature of the influence that health visitors wish to exercise and the nature of the policies they wish to affect. A policy can affect health favourably or adversely and, given that health is of value and worthy of achievement, then health visitors could only wish to support policies conducive to (people's) health and to challenge policies not conducive to health. The full implications of this principle then, are that health visitors seek to exert an influence on policies affecting people's health and that in applying this principle they will engage in political activity designed to support policies conducive to health and to challenge policies not conducive to health. However, it must be pointed out that it is not possible to influence policies, it is only possible to influence people, that is those who formulate the policies or carry them out.

6.6 At the macroscopic or national level, as members of a profession committed to health promotion, health visitors are in a position to exert an influence on policies affecting people's health. The professional bodies, by making representations to more powerful pressure groups, attempt to mobilize general public support for policies which will enhance standards of health care, and to highlight areas of potential difficulty arising in health care and social service provision. These professional bodies also submit evidence to Royal Commissions and to other working groups set up under the auspices of government to consider various aspects of health care policy. In this way they hope that influence on policy can be exerted. Also at the macroscopic level representatives of professional bodies are nominated to become members of these same groups investigating areas of health need. By such participation it is clear that the opportunity to influence policy is available to the profession.

6.7 M. Baly, in talking about the public service professions[5], suggests that they have an implied contract with society to give a service and are worthy of that contract on two grounds. Firstly, because they possess a body of knowledge and skills based upon a long period of training and society has need of these skills; and secondly, because the professions share a code of ethics which indicate how patients and clients should be served and the social attitudes that should be accepted. All nurses should accept the value of health; and, as outlined in the Royal College of Nursing discussion document on a code of professional conduct[6], this means that they have a responsibility to be concerned with political and social issues whenever they are relevant to the prevention of disease and the delivery of health care. The code of the International Council of Nurses[7] states "the nurse shares with other citizens the responsibility for initiating and supporting action to meet the health and social needs of the public".

6.8 That professions allied to health visiting see a need to influence Government policy is also evident, not only from literature relevant to nursing as outlined above, but also from literature relevant to social work. In the British Association of Social Work discussion paper on a code of ethics[8] it is stated that the social worker "has the right and duty to bring to the attention of those in power and of the general public ways in which the activities of government or society create or contribute to hardship or suffering or mitigate against their relief". That health visitors do seek to influence government policy is evident from the activity of their professional associations over the last few years. For example, in 1975 evidence was submitted to the Home Office on Marriage Guidance and to Parliamentary Select Committees on the Abortion (Amendment) Bill, on Violence in the Home and on Child Abuse and Preventive Medicine. Evidence was also submitted to the Department of Education and Science enquiry into Special Education and to the Jay Committee enquiring into Mental Handicap Nursing Care. At the request of the Department of Health and Social Security comments were sent on several draft discussion papers and circulars on matters including the sterilization of children under sixteen, neonatal care of babies and abortion counselling.

6.9 With regard to the opportunities for health visitors in general to influence the policies of governments and statutory bodies at local community level, it is more than likely that in their daily work individual health visitors seek to influence courses of action relevant to people's health either planned or carried out by local government departments, for example the Social Services Department, the Housing Department or the Education Department. They may seek to influence the Electricity Board or the Water Board. They may be acting on behalf of one particular individual or family or they may be acting on behalf of many. In all these activities, they may be acting as individuals or as a group of health visitors and this activity could be described as political.

6.10 Also at local community level, a great deal has been written about the management of the Health Service in recent years and it seems to be recognised that if the service is to be effective there must be participative management. Haywood[9] defines this as "a system which does not grudgingly permit but actively encourages the front line of staff to bring their experience and knowledge into the service of management". He also suggests that the controller of resources is dependent on the professional workers for information, but that not all of them are in such a strong position as the medical profession. Health visitors, nurses and those in the paramedical professions find this acknowledged sphere of competence narrower and their advice correspondingly more likely to be unsolicited or ignored. Since these are the people in face to face contact with clients, others in the organisation depend upon the information that they can provide. Within the reorganised health service, health visitors should be able to participate by being represented on Professional Advisory Committees, by being members of Health Care Planning Teams and by being in contact with the members of the Community Health Councils.

6.11 The Professional Advisory Committees on which there are health visitors, have been established at Regional and Area level and these committees are consulted before the important planning and allocation decisions are made. The Health Care Planning Teams exist at District level, are multidisciplinary and concentrate on planning services to meet particular needs. Although the composition of the team will be adjusted to particular situations it will possibly include a health visitor. As the function of the Health Care Planning Team is to assess needs in order to effect changes in the services provided, health visitors if they are members of these Teams have a very important part to play and could influence policy in a constructive and positive way.

6.12 With regard to the Community Health Councils, Owen thinks that their establishment is one of the most important aspects of Reorganisation. Many of the Councils appear to be concentrating on becoming well informed about the health needs of local populations and the degree to which local provision meets these needs. They have a right to ask for and receive information from Area Health Authorities, and in this respect it is important that information on the health needs of local populations should be available from the health visiting service.

6.13 Again at local community level, health visitors are members of Primary Health Care Teams and in a publication of the British Medical Association[10] the fundamental responsibility of these teams is stated as being to the individual in the community. Shared responsibility in decision-making is essential and can be achieved only if there is adequate communication. That communication is inadequate at present comes over clearly from the health visiting profession and emphasis is more on the communication between general practitioners and health visitors than between other members of the team. The association that a health visitor has with a general medical practice is described in a variety of ways such as 'attached', 'aligned', 'linked', 'in liaison with' but no agreed definition appears to exist as to what these terms mean. However, in all the literature on Primary Health Care Teams it is recognised that the health visitor is a member.

6.14 In the research by Gilmore et al[11] on the work of the nursing team in general practice, the assumption that the placing of staff in close proximity to one another will of itself result in better communication is strongly challenged. It is stated by the authors that in their opinion, for a team to work effectively, processes need to be developed for the application of organised effort in executing tasks. This involves communication, co-operation and co-ordination, and could perhaps be achieved by some degree of multi-disciplinary training.

6.15 In the publication of the Health Visitors Association 'Health Visiting in the Seventies'[12] it was pointed out that too few general practitioners understood the independent responsibility of health visitors. If they were unwilling to fulfil their functions as perceived by the G.P.s they were considered to be uncooperative. This was borne out by the research of Gilmore et al showing that health visitors were not well understood or appreciated by the doctors. The doctors were able to describe the role of the health visitors, but expressed doubts about the need for some of their activities, particularly in relation to primary prevention. There are strong arguments which support the inclusion of health visitors in Primary Health Care Teams; for it should provide a better service for the public because the health visitors could influence policies with their knowledge of individuals, families and the local community, together with their interest in primary prevention and the promotion of health.

6.16 As suggested earlier political behaviour of any sort can be seen as a particular type of social behaviour, in which case it is necessary to differentiate between that political behaviour of health visitors pertaining to Governments and statutory bodies, and that pertaining to other groups and individuals. For example, general medical practitioners are not employed directly either by central or local Governments nor by a statutory body, but they plan and carry out courses of action relevant to people's health. A health visitor might wish to influence a G.P.'s policy on behalf of one of his patients, either by supporting it or challenging it. Is this to be termed 'political activity'? Similarly, according to Dingwall health visiting may be thought of as "the enforcement of normal family life, an interlocking network of performances depicting a particular pattern of rights and obligations and where parts are at variance with this pattern, their task is to manipulate the situation as a whole to bring it into as close an accord with normality as possible"[12]. If this view of health visiting is correct then at the microscopic or family level this could be described as political activity designed to influence courses of action affecting normal (healthy?) family life.

6.17 An obvious consequence of influencing policies affecting health is that health visitors are contributing to social change. At the macroscopic level of activity this can be seen in the examples previously cited of the activities of the professional associations. Also whether or not Dingwall's perception of health visiting is correct, health visitors do seek to influence the courses of action of individuals at the microscopic level and in so doing again are an instrumental factor in effecting social change.

6.18 In the course of their work, health visitors attempt to influence young parents with a view to their adopting courses of action conducive to healthy living. They encourage parents to provide balanced diets and by obtaining acceptance of immunisation and participation in developmental screening they can be seen as directly contributing towards social change.

6.19 As part of their function within the School Health Service health visitors participate in identifying the health needs of the school population and more specifically in their teaching role they encourage children to recognise and to adopt positive health strategies. By teaching children about the benefits of personal and community hygiene they may be imparting knowledge which will in future years create pressure from the public for general environmental improvement. In this respect again they are contributing to social change.

6.20 Similarly health visitors assist young parents to plan their families in such a way as to foster family health and cohesion. In doing so their objective is to secure the well-being of family members but incidentally they may also be affecting the future size of the population.

6.21 At the local community level their contributions to social change can be seen in their encouragement of interaction between groups of parents with similar needs. In this way they are instrumental in the creation of action groups which in turn provide facilities such as play groups and toy libraries for children, day centres for the elderly or any other health facility for which there is a local need. They are also concerned about the adverse effects upon children of living in high-rise buildings or in other housing conditions which are detrimental to health. If health visitors seek to influence policies in these situations then again they are contributing to social change.

6.22 The degree of influence which health visitors have on their clients is difficult to measure. The requirement that they engage in work of this nature, however, is clearly spelled out in the objectives for training students,[13] the first of which states that one main aspect of the work is "the prevention of mental, physical or emotional ill-health or the alleviation of its consequences".

6.23 For the purpose of any further elaboration of this principle it is important to distinguish the three levels at which health visitors seek to influence policies affecting health. The national or macroscopic level is illustrated in the activities of the professional body collectively; the individual or microscopic level is illustrated in the activities of individual health visitors acting with or upon other individuals and families; finally the intermediate ('mediascopic'?) level, is illustrated in the activities of one or a group of health visitors acting at local or community level.

6.24 It is also important to differentiate between wishing to influence, seeking actively to influence, and being effective in influencing since certain questions arise from these differences. One question which might be asked is to what extent are health visitors effective in influencing policies? Depending on the answer to this, other questions follow. How is the effectiveness achieved or why is it prevented? In establishing a body of knowledge it is essential to ask the questions in the right order and "what do we mean?" comes before "how do we know?" In other words conceptual clarification must come before justification.

6.25 It is also important to distinguish what 'is' and what 'ought to be'. There is a difference between the positive statement that 'health visitors seek to influence . . .' which can be empirically verified or refuted and the normative statement that 'health visitors ought to seek to influence . . .' which as a matter of opinion or belief cannot be empirically tested, although it does follow logically from an acceptance of the value of health.

6.26 For example, if the vast majority of health visitors are in fact seeking to influence then it is unlikely that they would be doing so unless they thought they 'ought'. But if only a few are seeking to influence then although they might think they ought, the remainder might think otherwise and there is a discrepancy between what some health visitors are doing and what others are doing. Is this important? A body of knowledge consists of 'what is known to be true'; but the body of knowledge in any discipline is often 'frayed at the edges' as hypotheses are continually postulated, validated or refuted. This is of consequence to practitioners as well as to teachers and researchers.

6.27 The difference between 'is' and 'ought' principles or the difference between positive and normative statements is the difference between rational and irrational behaviour as seen by others. In washing their hands while attending women in childbirth, midwives were perhaps behaving irrationally in applying this principle until Semmelweiss conducted an empirical investigation and Lister demonstrated the reason scientifically. Then there was confluence between 'ought' and 'is'. Nevertheless, it remains important to differentiate conceptually what 'is' from what 'ought to be' since 'seeking to influence' presupposes a desire to be effective and raises many questions for research which are beyond the present terms of reference.

References

1. Duverger, M. (1967). The Idea of Politics. Methuen.
2. Owen, D. (1976). In Sickness and in Health. Quartet Books.
3. Raphael, D. (1976). Problems of Political Philosophy, p. 27–32. Revised edition Macmillan.
4. Open University. (1972). Health Decision Making in Britain V.
5. Baly, M. (1972). Professional Responsibility in the Community Health Services. HM & M.
6. Royal College of Nursing. (1976). Code of Professional Conduct (discussion document).

7. International Council of Nurses. (1973). Code for Nurses.
8. British Association of Social Work (1971). A Code of Ethics for Social Work. Discussion Paper 2.
9. Haywood, S. C. (1974). Managing the Health Service. George Allen & Unwin.
10. British Medical Association. (1974). Primary Health Care Teams.
11. Gilmore, M. et al. (1974). The Work of the Nursing Team in General Practice. C.E.T.H.V.
12. Dingwall, R. (1976). The Social Organisation of Health Visitor Training. Nursing Times Occasional Papers. February 19th 1976.
13. C.E.T.H.V. (1971). Handbook for Tutors and Examiners. (Second Edition).

Chapter 7

The Facilitation of Health-Enhancing Activities

7.1 This principle is considered to be applicable at individual, family and community level and is fundamental to the health visitor's role. The 'facilitation' or 'enabling' aspect of health visiting will be seen to operate at two distinct levels. First, at the client level where the health visitor seeks to facilitate some activity or behaviour desired in or by the client. This is normally achieved through counselling or health teaching activities. Second, at the colleague level where the intention is to facilitate activity within the health team (or related teams), for the benefit of the client or the client group. This latter intention may be achieved through communication and referral within the team so as to initiate planned activity on behalf of the client.

7.2 The wording of this principle was the subject of much debate as the noun 'facilitation' was thought to be inelegant and therefore not used in everyday speech. The substitution of the word 'planning' was considered but finally rejected as it was felt that this word implied direct activity and health visitors acting upon this principle could find themselves for example planning sport activities. 'Health Care' was also considered as a substitute for 'health enhancing activities' but the latter phrase was considered preferable as it has a wider connotation of which care is merely a part.

7.3 The concept of the health visitor as a facilitator is not new. In the Jameson Report (1956)[1] the health visitor was seen as "a common point of reference, a common source of information, a common adviser on health teaching, a common factor in family welfare".

7.4 The C.E.T.H.V. in 1967[2] published a statement outlining the concept of the function of the health visitor, which was to be a first step towards the publication of a fuller statement which gave the background to its training policy. The Working Party engaged in this task stated "If the Health Visitor is essentially concerned with the promotion and maintenance of good health, then it is essential that she should be able to identify the various factors which make for ill-health and so see how she can contribute to minimizing their influence. The health visitor has the opportunity to see where community resources are unavailable or where individuals are unable to use such resources as are present. In these circumstances, she may take the initiative in developing the necessary provision through co-operation with the appropriate department or colleagues. Thus she may be instrumental in seeing that play groups, child minders, children's play grounds, mothers' clubs, old people's clubs are adequate in her area and she will endeavour to see that individuals and families receive adequate financial help; she will do her best to ensure better conditions for the family. So, an important part of her function, in closest co-operation with others is concerned with ensuring that the individual receives adequate 'supplies', not only physical, but emotional, social and cultural, in order to develop healthily".

7.5 The report continued: "The health visitor has an important part to play in helping individuals and families to cope with those crises that inevitably occur in the best community and environmental conditions i.e. school entry, going to work, engagement, marriage, pregnancy, childbirth, the climacterium and retirement. All are likely to be associated with an increased chance of crises ... teachers, clergy and social workers are available to help people through these periods of possible crisis, but the health visitor should be able to give anticipatory guidance, warm support and if appropriate, practical help, so that the individual makes a good adaptation and emerges strengthened rather than weakened by the experience".

7.6 Three years later in 1970 in their evidence to the Committee on Nursing (Briggs),[3] the C.E.T.H.V., in discussing the future of health visiting stated, "Health visitors are already playing an important role in health centres and group practices, organising antenatal clinics for General Practitioners, carrying out health teaching and undertaking surveillance of vulnerable groups such as the elderly. It seems certain that this work will steadily expand and that the health visitor will become the main influence in promoting a much more preventive approach in general practice in the future ...

... She will continue to work with expectant mothers, and to visit all new births in the practice, surveying children under five and counselling on the many facets of child development and its implications. She will follow up patients discharged from hospital, and visit those suffering from long term illness cared for by the family, regardless of the need for nursing care. She is concerned with handicapped patients including the mentally subnormal some of whom will be under the care of another statutory service. There will in addition be other vulnerable groups as dictated by needs: for example, those recently bereaved or suffering from some special stress, and particular referrals to her from other agencies. . . .

A number of medical problems within a practice may be covered by the organisation of special clinics. These will include the traditional surveillance of the well child and of geriatric patients, and other special sessions to meet individual practice needs, i.e., clinics for the guidance of hypertensive or obese patients. The health visitor will take part in these clinics. . . .

In the clinic setting the health visitors' activities will include:

(a) consultation at baby and toddler clinics.

(b) conduct of health education to meet the health needs of the individual practice concerned. This might include work with expectant mothers, mothercraft classes, or the institution of a parent or teenage discussion group.

(c) attendance at antenatal sessions to begin contact with the families, giving health advice and in some cases making plans with the expectant mother for her confinement.

(d) the planning and organisation of geriatric clinics, arranging health education programmes and giving medico-social and health advice to those attending.

(e) encouraging participation in immunisation programmes. . . .

Although attached to general practice an essential part of the health visitor's role is the facilitating of a relationship between home and school. This will be of particular value when a child's progress is being assessed. She will also have a contribution to make to group health education carried out in school to various age groups and the Council are of the opinion that this is a continuing role".

7.7 The view of the health visitor as a facilitator is apparent in the following studies. The Court Committee (1976)[4] endorsed these views in relation to the health of the school child and the need to facilitate home/school links and communication between statutory bodies concerned with children's health, welfare and education.

7.8 Gilmore et al (1974)[5] in their study of the work of nursing teams in thirty-nine general practices found that less than a third of the general practitioners in the teams studied expressed interest in work involving them in liaison with social agencies. Dealing with the social problems of their patients and providing information on appropriate social help were regarded by a high proportion of the doctors as responsibilities that should be assumed by health visitors.

7.9 Skeet (1974)[6] commenting on a study of recently discharged hospital patients, highlighted the apparent lack of communication between hospital and community staff, and the lack of planning for the after care of such patients which resulted from this. One of the recommendations made as a result of this study was for the planning of after care in advance of patients' discharge dates, organised in conjunction with the patients' general practitioners and the staff of community services, so as to provide an unbroken service. It was further recommended that health visitors should be so deployed as to provide a routine counselling service for recently discharged hospital patients.

7.10 Planning 'health enhancing activities' or 'health care' may be seen to involve recognition by the health visitor that health, like life, is part of a dynamic process; it moves and changes in relation to factors such as age, conditions of life, and family and social relationships.

7.11 In tracing the constantly changing developments in health visiting from its inception in the mid-nineteenth century, it is apparent that it has always had a medical context and has approached health and health promotion from that setting. This is not surprising as health care systems in the Western world are dominated by medical value systems, linked to the image of health as 'absence of illness' and limited mainly to the physical aspect until the 1940s. Illich (1975)[7] contends that in Western technological society we continue to act on a medical model of health. It is commonly recognised that since 1948 the National Health Service grew larger and more expensive but failed to produce 'health'. Wilson (1976)[8] quotes examples of how a clinical model of health based on disease eradication as opposed to health enhancement produces dependency in patients and robs the individual of his personal responsibility and freedom of choice. He contends that health education as presently conceived by many people, is based on a medical model of health and its content is often, therefore, concerned with attacking bad habits.

7.12 The C.E.T.H.V.'s Syllabus of Training (1965) introduced psychological and sociological perspectives to the health visitors' educational programme, which is based on previous general nurse and midwifery or obstetric training. These perspectives have encouraged in health visitors a questioning theoretical and liberal approach to situations which differs from the essentially unquestioning and practical basic nurse training. Health visitors emerge from their educational programmes and return to work within the structure of the Area Health Authority/Board and find themselves in conflict situations. On the one hand, their medical and nursing colleagues and managers may appear to have little regard for the emphasis they have learned to place on social, emotional and cultural aspects of a given situation; while on the other hand, they may find that other professional colleagues such as social workers tend to convey the impression that their assessment of situations is based almost exclusively on physical and medical aspects. Clarke (1973)[9] discussing the sterotype of health visitors commonly held by general practitioners and social workers refutes the views that the emphasis of their visits is placed on physical aspects of care. They demonstrate how current training policy has influenced the health visitors' approach to their work. This was particularly noted in relation to improved interpersonal skills resulting in the discussion of a wide range of topics concerned with the emotional and social, as well as the physical aspects of health. Health visitors report that client perceptions of their role vary considerably and it is likely that the movement towards primary health care teams may be effective in helping clients to differentiate between the respective roles of members.

7.13 For the individual, a health care plan which is acceptable and comprehensible is most likely to be effective. As health visiting interventions are largely unsolicited by the consumer it follows that identification of health needs and plans for their solution must take account of prevailing individual and collective value systems. The aim will be to enable the individual or the family to identify and articulate their own health needs and thus to participate according to their needs and possibilities in the proposed health enhancing activity. This demonstrates the contemplative approach which is necessary. Having established the motivation of the individual towards improving his health status, the health visitor then considers what the person can do alone towards this end, what he can learn to do with help, what he cannot do and what specific help is needed, what specific resources are available and acceptable.

7.14 Nurse (1975)[10] calls this "The Enabling Process", with the emphasis on creating a situation where the client's own resources can be mobilised, where the client can be enabled to make a decision to take any action necessary—helping the person to help himself. The result may be the solution of the problem or the client learning to live with its continued existence. The health visitor in the counselling role attempts to create an enabling environment, but it is for the client to decide whether or not to accept help.

7.15 As health visitors' responsibilities for care extend over long periods of time and may involve many meetings and visits, it can be seen that the opportunities for counselling are many, in home or in clinic settings. How these opportunities are used will be determined to a great extent by the workload; and thus the need for planning is again demonstrated.

7.16 A participative approach is also necessary in order to ensure that there is an exchange of information between all persons involved in the plan at each stage of the process. As health and social problems vary in intensity and complexity and as an increasing number of different specialised workers may have to be involved, it can be seen that the health visitors' facilitating role as the person of first contact needs to be clearly articulated and widely publicised and reinforced. They should be able to make more explicit to an ever increasing number of people, the nature of the presenting problem and how it is expressed by the client. It is necessary to incorporate a progressive element in this kind of intervention. As already stated health, like life, is constantly changing and health care plans need to be modified accordingly. At all stages as elaborated in the previous chapter, communication and co-ordination are of utmost importance in order to ensure that continuity is achieved.

7.17 Several studies and evidence from health visitors themselves,* draw attention to the fact that although this role is recognised, deployment of health visitors does not always allow for it to be fully utilized. The findings so far highlight the difficulties for the professional worker whose primary task is to promote health. They also present a challenge to policy makers, educators and practitioners alike in an era when health care planning is changing more rapidly than at any time in history. It seems, therefore, clear that the concept of health visitors as 'facilitators of health enhancing activities' is implicit in statements made by C.E.T.H.V. about their role and function. It is also clear that the health visitors themselves see this as an important principle of their interventions and subsequent actions.

References

1. Ministry of Health, Department of Health Scotland and Department of Education. (1956). An Inquiry into Health Visiting. (Jameson Report) HMSO.
2. C.E.T.H.V. (1967). The Function of the Health Visitor in the U.K.
3. C.E.T.H.V. (1970). Evidence to the Committee on Nursing.
4. DHSS (1976). Fit for the Future. Cmmd. 6684 Vol. 1. HMSO.
5. Gilmore, M. Bruce, N. Hunt, M. (1974). The Work of the Nursing Team in General Practice. C.E.T.H.V.
6. Skeet, M. (1974). Home from Hospital. MacMillan Journals London.
7. Illich, I. (1975). Medical Nemesis. Calder & Boyars.
8. Wilson, M. (1976). Health Enhancement or Disease Eradication—Some Ethical Considerations. Vol. 14 No. 3. J. Inst. Health Education.
9. Clarke, J. (1973). A Family Visitor. RCN London.
10. Nurse, G. (1975). Counselling & the Nurse. HM & M Publishers.

*See previous references 1, 3, 4, 5, 6 and 9.

Chapter 8

Further Issues

8.1 The current search for the principles of health visiting had its origin in the doubts expressed by tutors over the teaching of "principles and practice". These doubts could very well have arisen from certain difficulties experienced by students, since if students are happy and satisfied with their education then presumably their teachers are also, and doubts do not arise. In other words, was something happening out there in the real world that brought about a discrepancy between the ideal and the reality? As is clear from earlier chapters many changes have occurred since health visiting began. The concepts of health and illness have changed, and no longer is everything quite so black and white as it was even in the 1950s. Our whole way of life has changed with extraordinary rapidity since the last war, and there have also been fundamental changes in the National Health Service.

8.2 From the discussions at Nottingham and Loughborough it seems that many health visitors are experiencing a degree of professional insecurity. What is the nature of this insecurity and could it possibly have anything to do with 'principles'?

8.3 Generally speaking health visiting consists of using the appropriate skills in the application of theory to practice. In Section V of the current syllabus one of the items to be taught is "theories and methods of health visiting practice". The theories and methods of any discipline should form the base of the educational programme for students, but whose theories and whose methods are to be taught? There are books on the principles of nutrition, books on the theories of sociology and psychology, books on epidemiology and on child development and so on. Health visitors can be seen to be applying the principles of nutrition and their knowledge of psychology. They can be seen to be applying their knowledge of child development. But what are these 'theories and methods of health visiting practice' that tutors are assumed to be teaching, that fieldwork teachers are assumed to be interpreting and that health visitors are assumed to be putting into practice? Does part of the solution to the current dilemmas of practice lie in the answer to this question?

8.4 Only the value of health and the four principles which derive from it have been examined in this document because these were the only matters on which there was a reasonable amount of agreement; or if there was not agreement at least the issues were reasonably clear-cut. But there is much more to health visiting than is embodied by these four principles. What is needed is a theoretical model of health visiting to which all tutors, fieldwork teachers and practitioners subscribe and which they can present to students. The concept that knowledge is 'frayed at the edges' is of little consequence to students; it is the core that is important and that provides the security for practice, although students may well benefit from looking at the 'frayed edge' since it is they who will be the fieldwork teachers and tutors of tomorrow.

8.5 Principles are applicable in all similar circumstances and are relatively unchanging. This means that whatever our visiting priorities may be we will continue to 'search for health needs' etc., because we consider health to be of value and worthy of achievement. That principles are relatively unchanging does not mean they are written for all time. Over the years society changes, people change, health needs change and even health visitors change. One principle or piece of knowledge may eventually be seen to be no longer valid and will be replaced by another which is more appropriate to the changed circumstances. Very few health visitors or tutors will have both the time and the inclination to carry on with this examination of principles and the clarification of concepts. If only some can and will write down their findings then the 'theories and methods of health visiting practice' will at least exist outside of the mind. It is regrettable that time, the very commodity so necessary for this purpose is becoming so scarce for students, practitioners and teachers alike.

8.6 Much of the literature relevant to health visiting is descriptive; there is very little which actually explains how to do health visiting. Whenever the word 'principles' is used in the literature there is little elaboration of theory or method. The principles are usually implied but they are rarely examined or made explicit. For this reason the 'theories and methods' taught can only be the theories and methods of individual tutors based upon their own personal experience.

8.7 This same lack of security in health visiting theory also poses a problem for practitioners who may ask "is what I'm doing the same as what everyone else is doing"? The problem is particularly acute for fieldwork teachers who have the explicitly stated responsibility of correlating theory with practice. "How can I correlate theory with practice for the student when neither of us seems to know what the theory is"?

8.8 The production of this document is only a first step. It must be followed by on-going thorough analysis of the principles of health visiting practice by individuals which must be published. Only in this way will a body of theory emerge.

8.9 The question is often asked "what is unique about health visitors"? The answer is that it lies in the combination of their specific areas of knowledge and particular skills which is unique; and that they are the only professional workers to visit 'normal' families with a view to the promotion of health and prevention of illness. Both of these statements are undoubtedly true, but there is a uniqueness which goes beyond this and which is frequently the subject of humour both within and without the profession. Much of the time health visitors are seen by others as 'doing nothing', but it is this so-called 'nothing', that is done by health visitors that constitutes 'health visiting'. It is also this planned apparent inactivity such as 'support' that is so difficult to explain to others.

8.10 We frequently accuse sociologists and other scientists of using jargon but we ourselves hide behind our own jargon. This is so easy to do since the jargon of health visitors consists of words in everyday use. What do we mean by 'social advice', 'support', 'care', 'counsel', 'acceptance', 'intervention', 'confidentiality' and so on? It is the explanation of these abstract concepts which we use that will in reality illustrate practice for students.

8.11 Experiences such as Nottingham and Loughborough can be so challenging, frustrating and exciting at one and the same time, because an exercise such as the search for principles requires the rigorous examination of an activity called 'health visiting'; and since 'health visiting' is essentially a mental process as opposed to a physical activity the analysis of such a process by those who actually do it necessitates considerable mind-searching, the very thought of which can be appalling. Is it beyond the bounds of possibility that a body of theory for health visiting can be established? If we do not at least make the effort then we shall continue to be something of an enigma to others, and not only to others but to ourselves; and is this not simply the two sides of the same coin anyway? That it is not beyond the bounds of possibility should be obvious to anyone who was at Nottingham and Loughborough or who participated in the work of a local group; but that it is a time-consuming, arduous and painful task is equally obvious. Nevertheless, the attempt must be made for if tutors, fieldwork teachers, practitioners and students are plagued by doubts the quality of service will be affected.

8.12 One particular dilemma in relation to practice that seems to concern practitioners, which is again ultimately related to principles, is "are we or are we not practitioners in our own right"? Perhaps Donald Hicks has already answered this once and for all by suggesting that none of us is. Health visitors are salaried employees of a statutory body and in this respect cannot possibly be practitioners in their own right. The pamphlet "The Function of the Health Visitor" (CETHV) offers an explanation by saying that health visitors detect cases of need on personal initiative as well as acting upon referrals. Even if they ever were, health visitors are no longer free agents with regard to detection and action for they operate within powerful constraints, not least of which are the expectations others have of the role of the health visitor.

8.13 The statement could also mean that health visitors are free to exercise their own judgements within their recognised spheres of activity and will accept responsibility for so doing. (Responsibility also goes with this freedom). Perhaps this particular dilemma is related to influencing policies at the micro-level, "will someone give me the authority to challenge those policies of colleagues in other professions which in my considered judgement are not in the best interests of my client"? It should not be necessary to make this plea since health visitors are members of primary health care teams and team work should imply agreed courses of action.

8.14 Another dilemma of practice related to the above seems to be the 'attachment' controversy. It would appear from the Loughborough discussions that many health visitors feel they were more effective when they were operating in geographically defined areas. This may or may not be so since 'effectiveness' in health visiting is difficult to define, but irrespective of proof attachment and effectiveness obviously pose problems. Again, is there a link with theory and principles here? Do some of the misunderstandings and breakdowns in communication derive from health visitors' lack of security in the knowledge base from which they work, not the knowledge of Sections I–IV of the present syllabus but of Section V "The Principles and Practice of Health Visiting"?

8.15 From this continuing appraisal of the basis of health visiting, it should be possible to plan a curriculum that can be seen to be rationally derived and ordered. By examining each principle in detail, the skills, attitudes and knowledge needed to implement it can be established. The rationale underlying the syllabus can be more clearly identified and its relevance to health visiting seen, since it is to this that it owes its derivation.

8.16 Moreover, it is likely that some skills, attitudes and knowledge will be necessary for accomplishing more than one principle. The frequency of such occurrences can be used as one criterion for ranking the material to be included in a syllabus. As more and more is demanded of health visitors in practice, a rational choice of priorities within their already inadequate period of education becomes more and more essential.

8.17 A great deal of the material produced at Nottingham, Loughborough and by local groups seems at first sight to have 'got lost in the wash'. What has happened to the concepts of 'availability' and 'universality'? If there are principles which have something to do with either of these concepts then further mind-searching might produce them. In what sense is the health visitor to be available? Similarly with 'universality'; is health visiting a worldwide activity, performed for all people under all circumstances? What do we really mean, and how should all these questions be answered?

References have not been cited in the text, but material relevant to this chapter can be found in:

Chater, S. (1975). Understanding Research in Nursing. WHO.
Dingwall, R. (1976). The Social Organisation of Health Visitor Training. Nursing Times.
Occasional Paper 19.2.76–11.3.76.
Gilmore, M. et al (1974). The Work of the Nursing Team in General Practice. C.E.T.H.V.
Health Visitors Association (1975). Health Visiting in the Seventies.
Hicks, D. (1976). Primary Health Care—Chapter 10. DHSS.
Luker, K. Adjusting to Being a Health Visitor. Nursing Times HV. Supplement 30.10.76.
O'Sullivan, S. (1976). Thoughts on the Course for Health Visitors. Nursing Times Occasional Paper 25.11.76.
Scottish National Nursing and Midwifery Consultative Committee (1976). A New Concept of Nursing. Nursing Times Occasional Papers April.

The Participative Process

Since the health visitor tutors' conference at Wansfell in April 1974, when the exercise of re-appraisal began, one aim has been to involve in this thinking as many health visitors as possible from throughout the United Kingdom. In the first instance the tutors were to consider their ideas on the basis of the regions represented at the Standing Conference of Representatives of Health Visitor Training Centres. When the Working Group was set up the membership comprised one representative selected from each region, two of the Council's professional advisers, together with members from the Education Committee of the C.E.T.H.V. The latter were Mrs. Margaret White, Senior Nursing Officer, Merton, Sutton and Wandsworth Area Health Authority, and Mrs. C. Thelma Wilson, Principal Lecturer in Social Policy and Social Administration, North East London Polytechnic. Each of these was able to offer a different view of health visitor education from that of the tutors. We are most grateful to them for their invaluable contributions, and particularly to Mrs. Wilson, who was the only non-health visitor member of the group.

When the Working Group had arrived at a certain stage in its deliberations it wished firstly to share ideas with other tutors; and secondly if this proved that the thinking was acceptable, to widen the discussion by including health visitors from the field and from management. The first step resulted in the Workshop for Health Visitor Tutors held at Nottingham in March 1976, which was attended by 50 health visitor tutors representative of all parts of the United Kingdom, at which much of the time was spent in group work.

An account of this Workshop was produced to be used by the participants as a basis for further discussion. In the event, by March 1977, 450 copies had been sold, in addition to those circulated to participants.

The next stage was the formation of small geographically-determined and task-orientated groups, mostly initiated by tutors who had attended the Nottingham Workshop. Area Nursing Officers, and the Professional Organisations were informed of this development, and various grades of health visiting staff were involved on a voluntary basis. Inevitably there were some parts of the country which had not been represented at Nottingham, and where it was not so easy to obtain participation. However, a number of groups met during the summer and autumn of 1976 and sent in reports of their discussions and thinking which later provided the basis for the document used at the next Workshop at Loughborough.

Reports were prepared by the following groups:
Barnet
Bolton
Cambridge including Saffron Waldron, and Peterborough
Derbyshire
Edinburgh
Epping, including Harlow and East and West Rodings
Essex, Redbridge and Waltham Forest
Hereford, Worcester and Gloucester
Huddersfield
Luton
Manchester, including Tameside, Stockport and Trafford
Merton, Sutton and Wandsworth
North London, including Enfield, Tower Hamlets, Barnet and Camden
Northern Ireland
Nottingham
Reading
St. Albans
Slough
South Wales
Stevenage, groups from Bedfordshire, Northants, Buckinghamshire and Hertfordshire
Surrey University.

Other groups met for discussions, but did not actually send in written reports. Many health visitors have given much of their spare time and energies in contributing to this work.

The Workshop at Loughborough University in January 1977 was attended by 68 health visitors in addition to the members of the Working Group. It is interesting to note that the breakdown of attendance shows a representation of all grades of staff—so that each discussion group included practising health visitors, health visitor tutors and nursing officers.

Participants categorised by field of work

Director—Council for the Education and Training of Health Visitors
Health Visitor Tutors—28

Health Visitors—9
Fieldwork Teachers—10
Nursing Officers—5
Senior Nursing Officers—4
Divisional Nursing Officers—4
District Nursing Officers—1
Area Nurses Child Health—4
Area Nursing Officers—2
Geographical representation was also extensive as follows:
Scotland—3
Northern Ireland—5
Northern England—16
Midlands and East Anglia—16
Greater London Area—17
South England—10

A number of those attending came in their free time and paid their own expenses, but others were supported by Health Authorities, or by professional organisations at local or national level. All are warmly thanked, whether they have given their support by allowing members of their staffs time off and expenses, or whether they have given of their own time and money to undertake this task.

The Consultative Document

Following the Conference the Working Group has compiled this report, based on the ideas and thoughts forthcoming from the whole process of participation. Other work has been started which has not been included at this stage, but which will be of great use in any revision of the syllabus in the future.

The on-going exercise

Many of the geographical groups are continuing to follow-up ideas from the Loughborough Workshop, and it is hoped that they will meet to consider and comment on this Report.

Miss R. Schröck, a Lecturer in the Department of Nursing Studies, University of Edinburgh, was invited to join the Working Group at their first working week-end session. She subsequently joined the two workshops at Nottingham and Loughborough.

The members of the Working Group are grateful to Miss Schrock for her interest and involvement in the task of re-appraising the principles and practice of health visiting.

Miss Schrock's leadership and clarity of thought were of great benefit to members of the workshops when she led the plenary sessions. Through her analysis of the work of the small groups, she enabled the participants to perceive relationships in the material which were not previously obvious.

The Ongoing Process of Reappraisal

An edited version of the paper by Miss Schrock

The beginning of the process is very important. It illustrates the start of all those activities which, although called by various names, have a common denominator in the endeavour to reappraise, eg., research, conceptual revision, theory construction, examination of principles or even ideological reassessment.

The first two steps in this process are:

1 Established practices and explanations are being questioned by the practitioner.

2 Questioning arises out of the realisation that the established practices no longer seem to:

   (a) fulfil the demands made on the practitioner by the client or consumer (or by the material)

   (b) provide the practitioner with a measure that he/she is operating satisfactorily or efficiently and that current explanations for these practices no longer help to:

   (i) order and predict events with any certainty

   (ii) provide an acceptable rationale for practice.

This state of affairs is often experienced as a scientific or professional crisis. Suddenly, it seems, the old concepts and modes of thinking which appeared to have provided a perfectly satisfactory basis for a particular scientific or professional activity, are not only inadequate but also strangely uncertain. The dilemma experienced by people in such situations is almost bizarre.

No one would doubt that there is a group of people called health visitors. They exist, they carry out observable activities which can be described and categorised and compared with the activities of other people. These are matters of fact, open to verification. But, at the same time, the strange question arises whether in fact there is such a thing as health visiting. What has happened?

To emphasise the point: no one would deny that there are people who call themselves health visitors. We can count them, classify them by age or sex, describe their work and their clinets and so on. But this does not answer the question whether there is such a cognitive, conceptual entity which we can call health visiting as distinct from similar but other entities. So what we are encountering here is a conceptual problem.

To find the answer we would waste time, if we tried to learn more about health visitors, or about their work as it can be seen to be done, or about the things which they learn in the course of their training and education. We must focus our attention on the criteria in virtue of which we say that all these factual phenomena can be conceptualised under the term 'health visiting'. We must find out the rules in terms of which expressions are correctly or incorrectly used and we must particularly attend to the reasons which these criteria and rules embody, i.e. why we should draw one distinction rather than another, why we should characterise actions in one way and not in some different way.

That the participants at the 1974 Wansfell Conference were not in need of more factual information about health visiting or about health visitors was poignantly indicated by the statement:

> It was not easy to clarify the principles of health visiting except that they appeared to be expressed in ethical terms and shared with other caring professions. The conference ended with tutors questioning whether there were principles more specific to health visiting.

At this point the third step and the fourth in the process of reappraisal had been reached:

3 Uncertainty is experienced by the practitioner not only about various concrete aspects of his/her activity, but about its whole purpose or meaning.

4 Formerly specific aspects or variables have lost their specifity and have become diffuse by escaping precise definition.

It is at this stage that one must realise that the only solution lies in abandoning, at least for the time being, any attempt to add to, to refine or to rearrange the specifics, both the factual and conceptual content.

Whether this realisation and the resoluteness required to translate it into action is always allowed to become fully conscious, is a fascinating but also a crucial question. Particularly in all those human activities where time seems to be pressing in one way or another or where the demands on the practitioner are uninterrupted or even increasing, the above demand seems impossible. To abandon, even temporarily, the conceptual structures which so far have given a modicum of security during a process which by itself generates uncertainty, demands a great deal of courage. Or, to put it another way, to solve the increasing uncertainty, one must first create even more, and perhaps deliberately, total uncertainty! This is, as one may appreciate, a rather frightening prospect both for the individual and the group.

But this is the fifth step in the process of reappraisal:

5 By questioning the fundamental assumptions underlying the practice of the explanations, an even greater degree of uncertainty is created.

This, however, is what occurred during the early meetings of the Working Group which had been set up in 1975.

It may have been a fortunate coincidence and indeed, may not have been seen at the time to be a positive factor, that in asking me to contribute to the deliberations, a further source of creating more uncertainty was introduced into the process. The uninhibited questioning of some fundamental assumptions underlying the practice of health visiting was necessary, since these were meaningless unless the criteria for using them were spelt out in minute detail. It soon became apparent that what had once been a fairly effective framework for all these activities which we call health visiting had become insufficiently wide or flexible to accommodate all the developments which had taken place over the last twenty years. The next steps in the process are:

6 Reconstruction which starts with the identification and analysis of key concepts relevant to the practice under scrutiny.

7 Before these key concepts can be reorganised into a new, more effective conceptual framework, the field of conceptual enquiry must be extended in two ways:

(a) the use and meaning of these very same concepts must be examined in any other area where they appear to be of significance and their meaning and relationship in these other areas must be analysed.

(b) related 'questions' or 'problems' must be identified and reduced to the concept which is being 'questioned' or which proves 'problematical' so that these concepts can be incorporated into the continuing process of reappraisal.

This latter activity occupied much of the participants' time and effort during the days of the Nottingham Workshop. It alternated and was inter-related with what one must call the stage of 'experimenting with parts of a usable model'.

8 Conceptual and paradigmatic experimentation involves trying out and usually partly accepting and partly discarding various elements. This stage of experimentation must attempt to test any suggested solutions (or parts of a solution) for

(a) inherent consistency (informal logic)

(b) its explanatory value and power of the practice under scrutiny.

There is a danger that this phase can be prolonged and extended to such a degree that it becomes more and more difficult to correlate what is happening. Therefore the next step must be attempted, even tentatively, to keep control over the process:

9 Definitions and paradigms must be formulated and must be used to incorporate any new elements and any new part solutions.

There is a possibility that a point is reached where the attempted definition and the provisional paradigm or the set of principles prove unworkable. This, however, does not mean that a start from the very beginning has to be made. If a careful record of the criteria and rules expressed in these conceptual structures has been kept, it can fairly easily be seen in what way the solution so far attempted is still valid and in what specific way it has to be modified.

The next stages can be summarised in the last three steps:

10 Conclusive conceptual and paradigmatic statements must be made.

11 The specific question/problem which started off the process of reappraisal must be answered/solved.

12 The 'new' concept/model/set of principles/theory must be shared with all practitioners and must be tested in its application to the practical endeavour under scrutiny.

However, the twelfth step should not literally come 'at the end' but the whole development of the process of reappraisal should be shared to the greatest possible extent with the practitioner.